Men'sHealth

TODAY 20 08

Men'sHealth

TODAY 2008

YOUR BEST LIFE STARTS

NOW

RODALE

© 2008 by Rodale Inc.
Interior photographs
Page xi by Beth Bischoff; page 41 by Digital Vision/Getty Images;
page 75 by Ondrea Barbe; page 103 by Michael Blann/Getty Images;
page 153 by Ken Anderson; page 213 by Christopher Robbins/Getty Images;
page 265 by Indeed/Getty Images; page 317 by Daniel Garriga

Printed in the United States of America
Rodale Inc. makes every effort to use acid-free ⊗, recycled paper ♲.

Book design by Susan Eugster

Library of Congress Cataloging-in-Publication Data

ISBN 13 978–1–59486–696–8
ISBN 10 1–59486–696–1

2 4 6 8 10 9 7 5 3 1 hardcover

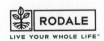

LIVE YOUR WHOLE LIFE™

We inspire and enable people to improve their lives and the world around them

For more of our products visit **rodalestore.com** or call 800-848-4735

CONTENTS

INTRODUCTION

Do you feel it? It's time to make a change. We know this because you're holding in your hands a powerful tool, one that will motivate you to look, feel, and be your best ever.

After all, who doesn't want to be the best? And in pursuit of that, this book offers pages and pages of advice to help you *look* your best ever. You'll fight fat with the Thinking Man's Diet and uncover your abs with the Abs Diet Arsenal. Get fit with the Statutes of Stretching and the Ever-Evolving Workout. Choose more carefully what you put into your mouth with Leaner Cuisines and Perfect Foods. Put together your best look with the Color Advantage and some simple Image Upgrades.

Of course, looking your best means little if you don't *feel* your best. Read on to gain Maximum Immunity, some Infection Protection, and Crazy Cures for all sorts of nagging ailments. This is the place to look for simple solutions to life's everyday headaches. But if it's the big stuff that's worrying you, cheat death by learning about the Skin Cancer Epidemic. Get some insurance for your ticker with Your Winning Numbers and Heart Smarts. And glimpse the future of health care by going behind Medicine's Front Line.

It's our hope that once you look and feel your best, you'll *be* the best ever. What does that mean to you? Perhaps you want to be the best father. Learn to Parent Better to be More Than Just the Ugly Mom and from reading stories about other dads in My Unexpected Children and My Summer of Strength. Or perhaps you want to be the best at whatever you do forty, fifty, sixty, plus hours a week on the job. You'll learn to Work Smarter by following our Promotion Plan, taking a look into the Mentor Mirror, and heeding the Firing-Squad Survival Guide.

You've already taken the first step toward the best you, ever. Now take the next one—turn the page.

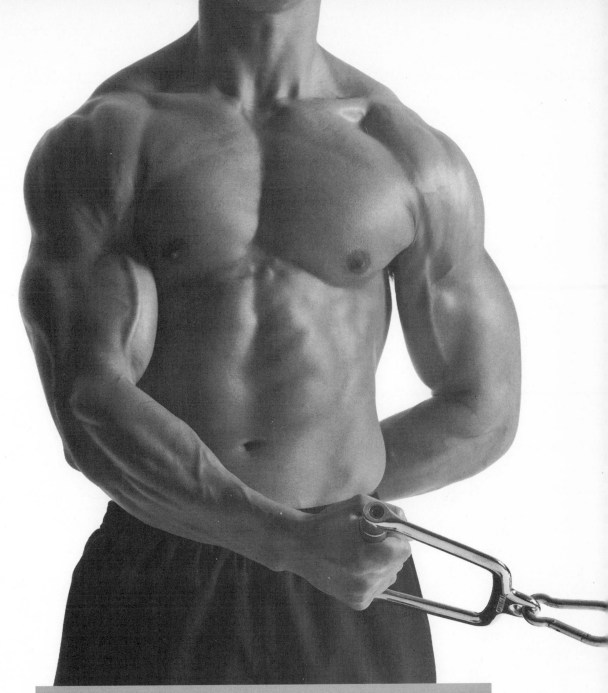

PART ONE
FIGHT FAT

THE THINKING MAN'S DIET

AVOID THE FIVE LEADING WEIGHT-LOSS PITFALLS FOR MEN

BY DAVID SCHIPPER

In prehistoric times, you would have emerged from a cave to survey the landscape for food. For survival, your brain would have urged devouring anything you could kill or uproot. Yet, when you weren't out hunting sloths, you would have become one for similar reasons. "When we didn't need to get food, we saved energy," says Paul M. Thompson, MD, director of the preventive-cardiology program and of cardiovascular research at Hartford Hospital in Connecticut. "That was how you survived; you didn't waste energy."

See how that survival hardwiring would be a one-way ticket to a blubber belly today? Whether you're in a supermarket or a restaurant, your brain still tells you to eat whatever you can lay your hands on. Once you've filled your stomach, it still seduces you into kicking back, a decision made easier by Barcaloungers and big-screen TVs. So in the deepest recesses of your noggin, dieting and burning off pounds will need to override 40,000 years of evolutionary programming.

What will your brain do when you ask it to betray itself? Here are the five dieting traps most likely to trip you—and ways to avoid them.

PITFALL 1:
SOCIAL SITUATIONS

"Our patients talk about people pressuring them to eat because they think they're not enjoying themselves," says Martin Binks, PhD, director of behavioral health at the Duke Diet and Fitness Center. Plus, men are expected to eat up, having been raised to equate manhood with a big appetite, adds Lisa Dorfman, PhD, RD, a licensed psychotherapist and a spokeswoman for the American Dietetic Association.

HOW TO AVOID IT: Have your comeback ready: "I can't eat because I had a big meal an hour or so before I got here." Or, "After I leave here, I have a date with an amazing woman I just met, so I don't want to fill up here first."

BONUS TIP: Nibble on appetizers like you'd sip a cocktail. Others will see that you're holding something, derailing the "Why aren't you eating?" issue. Plus, you'll feel fuller.

PITFALL 2:
SABOTAGE BY YOUR WIFE OR GIRLFRIEND

When you shape up, your better half suddenly has a choice: Undertake a transformation of her own, or inadvertently sabotage yours. Many times she'll choose the latter, often subconsciously. After all, the better you look, the more other women will be checking you out. "'Sabotage' is a very strong word, but she really will ask you to go to the store more often for cookies and other things she wants," says Valerie Berkowitz, MS, RD, a nutritionist at the Center for Balanced Health in New York City. "It's a sign that she misses your old life, the one where you always ate bad food together and had fun doing so."

HOW TO AVOID IT: Compromise. "If she insists on going out for pizza, have a few slices each instead of polishing off an entire pie," says Christopher Mohr, PhD, RD, whose doctoral research focused on behavioral weight loss.

BONUS TIP: "Include her by suggesting that she work out with you," says Dr. Mohr. "Find mutually enjoyable activities, so it doesn't come across as 'You're fat, so work out.'"

PITFALL 3:
THINKING YOU'RE THINNER THAN YOU REALLY ARE

After interviewing thousands of people, a team of Dartmouth brain researchers led by Putnam Keller, PhD, determined that women use anxiety and fear to help them reach goals. So they count calories and stick with gym schedules. Men, on the other hand, rely more on hope, which makes it harder for them to stick with diets. "Hope seduces men into mentally enjoying a desired future in the here and now before attaining it," says Dr. Keller. This keeps us from sacrificing.

HOW TO AVOID IT: Take a picture. Two-thirds of adult Americans are overweight, yet only 40 percent believe themselves to be too fat. "When people think of obesity, they think of the extremely obese, like 400 pounds or so," says Kimberly Truesdale, PhD, lead author of a University of North Carolina study that found that only 15 percent of obese adults recognize how heavy they are. "Your reflection in a mirror won't always register in your brain, but a picture will," says Berkowitz.

BONUS TIP: More than three-quarters of successful dieters cite a single emotional or physical incident that prompted them to get healthy, according to the National Weight Control Registry. Recognize yours when it comes.

PITFALL 4:
LETTING STRESS GET THE BEST OF YOU

Stressed-out guys are more likely to binge eat because of a brain hormone called corticotrophin-releasing factor (CRF), according to Georgetown University researchers. The study, published in the journal *BMC Biology*, found that when rats' brains have levels of CRF comparable to amounts found in stressed humans, the rodents' cravings for sugary treats and other rewards triple. "This traps individuals into chasing incentives they could normally resist," the study authors say.

HOW TO AVOID IT: Breathe more slowly and deliberately. "Use breathing to interrupt unhealthy thoughts before they become reality, so you give yourself a window of choice," says Grant Sutherland, APHP, a licensed hypnotist and founder of SlimClinic, a division of Keystone

Wellness, which specializes in emotional eating and obesity. Feel a binge coming on? Focus on the center of your chest and, for 1 minute, make your inhalations and exhalations last 5 seconds apiece, which will slow you down. It might sound simplistic, but it actually works. "Your breathing will cause your mind to relax, no matter how stressed your body is," Sutherland advises.

BONUS TIP: Sit next to Natalie Portman, or at least imagine her at your side. Chances are you'll eat with better manners (and hence more slowly) than if you were sitting on the sofa in your boxer shorts.

PITFALL 5:
BEING A PERFECTIONIST

An all-or-nothing approach to weight loss is a prescription for disaster. "We feel so completely defeated when we fail that it can take us away from the plan entirely," says Warren Huberman, PhD, a clinical psychologist at the New York University school of medicine who works with patients through the university's program for surgical weight loss.

HOW TO AVOID IT: Make dieting seem less onerous by giving yourself permission to slack off once in a while. Berkowitz suggests allowing one-fifth of your consumption to come from nondiet foods. This means you can cheat every fifth meal each day, or cheat all day every fifth day—whichever option fits best with your lifestyle. "If you're doing a good job of sticking to your diet, let the foods you're craving be a reward by scheduling them into a meal," says Joshua Klapow, PhD, a psychologist at the University of Alabama at Birmingham.

BONUS TIP: Ask yourself what you'll look and feel like 5 years down the road, and how that will affect your family. Then write out your answers. "Motivation levels go way up when you do that," says Klapow.

LEANER CUISINES

LOSE WEIGHT WITH THESE SEVEN FAT-FIGHTING MEALS FROM AROUND THE GLOBE

BY DEVIN ALEXANDER

No matter what you order at a restaurant, they always hear, "Make it extra-heavy on the carbs and fat." After all, restaurateurs are concerned about their bottom lines, not your waistline. And whether it's Italian or Mexican, Chinese or Greek, piling plates high with inexpensive pasta, rice, and bread—along with loads of butter—is a smart business tactic. It ensures that you feel you're getting your money's worth, without eating into the company profits. The only loser in this relationship? Your flab-covered abs.

We offer this alternative: fat-fighting meals from around the world that you can make in your own kitchen. The secret isn't tiny, Frenchman-like portions; it's a redistribution of nutrients. That's because we've stripped away the empty calories—scaling back unnecessary starches and fats—and infused each meal with more belly-filling fiber and metabolism-boosting protein. The result is a weeklong, international menu that's anything but fattening—or boring. The bonus? No tipping required.

HOW TO USE THESE RECIPES

Each recipe makes one serving. So if you're having company or want leftovers, simply multiply the ingredients by the total number of desired servings. To make cleanup easy, preheat your skillet and lightly coat it with olive-oil spray before cooking. For convenience, we've suggested specific brands of some products. However, you can substitute the brand of your choice, as long as you keep the serving size consistent.

ITALIAN

SAUSAGE-AND-PEPPER PASTA

½ cup Barilla Plus rotini pasta

5 ounces Italian turkey sausage (casing removed)

½ medium yellow bell pepper, cut into strips

½ medium red bell pepper, cut into strips

¾ cup Classico Italian Sausage with Peppers & Onions marinara sauce

2 teaspoons reduced-fat grated Parmesan

As you cook the pasta according to the package directions, spray a medium nonstick skillet with olive-oil spray and place it over medium-high heat. When the pan is hot, add the sausage and cook until browned, breaking it apart to create meaty bites. Add the peppers and cook until they're just tender and the sausage is no longer pink. Pour the sauce into the pan and stir the ingredients together. When the mixture is hot (about 2 minutes), stir in the pasta. Transfer it to a bowl, and top with Parmesan.

MAKES 1 SERVING

PER SERVING: 497 CALORIES, 39 G PROTEIN, 52 G CARBOHYDRATES, 15 G FAT (3 G SATURATED), 8 G FIBER

MEXICAN

STEAK-AND-BEAN BURRITO

1 Mission Carb Balance 10" tortilla

1 teaspoon burrito seasoning

5 ounces top round steak, cut into thin strips

¼ cup canned fat-free refried beans

1 tablespoon sour cream

¼ cup 2%-fat Mexican-blend cheese

½ cup chopped romaine lettuce

½ cup pico de gallo, drained

1 tablespoon taco sauce

Preheat the oven to 400°F, wrap the tortilla in foil, and place it in the oven. Mix the burrito seasoning with the steak to coat the meat, then place it in a nonstick skillet over medium heat. Brown the steak on both sides.

Meanwhile, warm the refried beans in the micro-wave on low in 20-second intervals until hot. Unwrap the tortilla and spread sour cream down the center, leaving 1" bare on both ends. Spoon the beans over the sour cream, followed by the steak, cheese, lettuce, pico de gallo, and taco sauce. Fold in the bare margins of the tortilla, then fold in one side and roll the tortilla until all the edges are down.

PERCENTAGE OF MEN WHO WOULD RATHER GET DIVORCED THAN BE OVERWEIGHT:
30

MAKES 1 SERVING

PER SERVING: 547 CALORIES, 51 G PROTEIN, 55 G CARBOHYDRATES, 18 G FAT (8 G SATURATED), 25 G FIBER

CHINESE

PORK FRIED RICE

2 teaspoons toasted sesame oil

4 ounces pork top loin chop, cut into thin strips

½ cup chopped onion

1 cup cooked Uncle Ben's microwavable brown rice

¼ cup frozen peas

2 egg whites

1 tablespoon hoisin sauce

2 teaspoons low-sodium soy sauce

Place a large nonstick skillet over medium-high heat and add 1 teaspoon of the oil, along with the pork and onion. Cook until the pork is no longer pink inside, then place the meat on a plate. Add the rice, peas, and remaining oil to the onion in the pan. Stir-fry for 2 minutes, then push it to the sides. Coat the exposed area with olive-oil spray and add the egg whites. Mix into the rice and continue to cook for another 2 to 3 minutes, until the egg is cooked. Stir the pork mixture into the rice, then add the hoisin and soy sauces. Cook until hot.

MAKES 1 SERVING

PER SERVING: 579 CALORIES, 42 G PROTEIN, 69 G CARBOHYDRATES, 15 G FAT (3 G SATURATED), 7 G FIBER

CAJUN

CAJUN CHICKEN FINGERS AND SWEET-POTATO FRIES

1 medium sweet potato, peeled and cut into sticks about ¼" thick

2 teaspoons extra-virgin olive oil

1 teaspoon (or more) Cajun seasoning or rub

6 ounces boneless, skinless chicken breasts, cut into strips

Ketchup (optional)

Creole mustard (optional)

Preheat the grill to high heat and the oven to 450°F. Toss the sweet-potato sticks in 1 teaspoon of the oil and ½ teaspoon of Cajun seasoning. Place them in a single layer on a nonstick baking sheet so they don't touch each other. Bake the fries for 10 minutes, flip them over, and bake for an additional 10 to 15 minutes, or until they're tender and starting to brown. Meanwhile, toss the chicken in the remaining oil, then sprinkle with Cajun seasoning. About 5 minutes before the fries are done, grill the chicken for about 2 to 3 minutes per side, or until the strips are no longer pink inside. Serve immediately with ketchup and Creole mustard, if desired.

MAKES 1 SERVING

PER SERVING: 475 CALORIES, 42 G PROTEIN, 55 G CARBOHYDRATES,
10 G FAT (1 G SATURATED), 8 G FIBER

INDIAN

CURRIED SHRIMP KEBABS WITH BASMATI RICE

½ cup basmati rice

6 ounces peeled medium shrimp

8 cherry tomatoes

8 1"-square pieces red onion (1 layer only)

1 teaspoon curry paste

½ tablespoon extra-virgin olive oil

2 skewers

Preheat the grill to high heat. Meanwhile, cook the rice according to the package directions. Then, in a medium bowl, combine the shrimp, tomatoes, onion, curry paste, and oil. Skewer the shrimp, tomatoes, and onion, alternating among them. Turn the grill to low and place the skewers side-by-side across it. Grill them for about 3 to 4 minutes per side, until the shrimp have plumped. Serve over the rice.

MAKES 1 SERVING

PER SERVING: 463 CALORIES, 40 G PROTEIN, 44 G CARBOHYDRATES, 14 G FAT (2 G SATURATED), 5 G FIBER

GREEK

BROILED LAMB CHOP OVER TOMATO-CUCUMBER SALAD

2 medium tomatoes
½ medium cucumber
6 ounces boneless leg-of-lamb chop
½ teaspoon extra-virgin olive oil
½ teaspoon garlic paste
Salt
Pepper
1 cup microwavable frozen spinach
⅓ cup finely chopped red onion
1 tablespoon Greek vinaigrette
¼ cup crumbled reduced-fat feta cheese

Preheat the grill to high heat. Cut the tomatoes in quarters across the stem; slice the piece of cucumber in half lengthwise, then cut into ¼" pieces. For both, use a spoon to scrape out and discard the seeds, then place the vegetables in a medium bowl. Rub the lamb on all sides with the oil and garlic paste, and season with salt and pepper. Grill for about 3 to 4 minutes on each side, or until the meat reaches the desired doneness. Remove the lamb from the grill and let it sit for 5 minutes. While the lamb sits, microwave the spinach according to the package directions. Then add the onion, vinaigrette, and 2 tablespoons of the feta to the tomato-and-cucumber mixture. Toss the ingredients together, then spoon them onto the center of a dinner plate. Cutting against the grain, slice the lamb into thin strips and place them on the salad. Sprinkle the remaining feta over the top and serve with the spinach on the side.

MAKES 1 SERVING

PER SERVING: 521 CALORIES, 53 G PROTEIN, 36 G CARBOHYDRATES, 20 G FAT (6 G SATURATED), 11 G FIBER

JAPANESE

TERIYAKI SALMON BOWL WITH BROCCOLI

6-ounce boneless salmon fillet
2½ tablespoons honey teriyaki sauce
½ cup microwavable frozen broccoli
½ cup Uncle Ben's microwavable brown rice

Preheat the grill to high heat. Spray a sheet of foil about four times the size of the salmon with olive-oil spray. Rub the salmon with ½ tablespoon of the teriyaki sauce. Place the foil on a grill rack, then place the salmon on the foil. Grill for about 5 minutes per side, or until the salmon is light pink and no longer shiny throughout. Microwave the broccoli and rice according to the package directions. Place the rice in a medium-size shallow bowl. Top with the salmon, then add the broccoli around the fish. Drizzle the remaining sauce over the top.

MAKES 1 SERVING

PER SERVING: 519 CALORIES, 41 G PROTEIN, 44 G CARBOHYDRATES, 20 G FAT (4 G SATURATED), 5 G FIBER

THE ABS DIET ARSENAL

ENJOY THESE 6-MINUTE MEALS FOR SIX-PACK ABS

BY DAVID ZINCZENKO

A lot can happen in 6 minutes. It's enough time to make or break a job interview, have great sex, or listen to all of Quiet Riot's greatest hits.

And in 6 minutes, you can find your six-pack abs.

Not with a CAT scan or an endoscope or a self-powered liposuction machine, but with an intelligent, well-balanced, and (most of all) easy eating plan made up of great-tasting foods. Not a fad diet. And no weird vacuum-sealed meals that have to be special-delivered to your home by the food police. Just sensible food that's fast and easy—and isn't pushed through your car window by a guy in a paper hat.

Abs, after all, aren't made in the gym; they're made in the kitchen. What you put into your mouth is far more important than what you put into your workout. For example, in an analysis of 33 clinical trials, Brazilian researchers determined that diet controls about 75 percent of weight loss. Of course, that doesn't mean exercise isn't an important part of the fat-burning formula. But if you want the fastest results, a smart eating plan is the foundation of your gut-busting program.

So that's why we're introducing the Abs Diet Arsenal: easy guidelines that can make you lean for life. They're based on my book *The Abs Diet*, which has guided more than a million people in making permanent changes in their food intake and fat output.

Too many diets are about rules and deprivation. And let's face it: Once you're told you can't have something, don't you just want it more? So I want you to stop thinking you have rules. I simply want you to rethink the way you eat. Follow the guidelines below, and you'll feel what it's like to eat right, stay satisfied, and fuel your body with high-octane energy.

Because I believe abs, beer, and *Star Wars* movies aren't the only good things that come in sixes, I've developed six guidelines for the Abs Diet. Eat this way and you'll be able to ditch the old rules—as well as your old body.

GUIDELINE 1

OLD DIETS: Eat breakfast, lunch, and dinner.

ABS DIET: Eat six times a day.

Old diet systems ensure that you stay hungry by forcing you to eat a daily calorie count that's lower than Jessica Simpson's SAT scores. I don't want you hungry; I want you full. When you're full, you won't be as tempted (or likely) to steamroll your way through pizza boxes. And the way you'll get full is by eating six times a day, choosing from the nutritional heroes you'll meet below. By eating every few hours, you'll keep your metabolism revved and ensure overall stomach satisfaction. The great thing about the Abs Diet powerfoods is that, because they're high in nutrients, protein, healthy fats, and fiber, they make it almost impossible to overeat. Proper nutrition will leave you feeling satiated all day long.

HOW TO DO IT: Eat three standard meals and three smaller snacks. For example:

8:00 a.m.	Breakfast
11:00 a.m.	Snack
1:00 p.m.	Lunch
4:00 p.m.	Snack
6:00 p.m.	Dinner
9:00 p.m.	Snack

GUIDELINE 2

OLD DIETS: Deprive yourself of specific foods.

ABS DIET: Indulge in specific foods—the Abs Diet Power 12.

Most diets treat you as if you're the kid and they're the parent: No this, no that, no fruit, no bread, no meat, no potatoes, no sugar, no, no, no, no. And you end up hearing "no" more often than the science-club president 3 weeks before the prom. Yes, it's true that there are foods and substances so toxic that you should stiff-arm them like Reggie Bush shaking off a tackle. But there's an enormous world of wonderful foods out there just waiting for you. And it's not all veggies and tofu; the preferred foods are as diverse in taste as in nutritional power. How convenient that they line up next to the letters in ABS DIET POWER:

A	Almonds (and other nuts)
B	Beans (and other legumes)
S	Spinach (and other green vegetables)
D	Dairy
I	Instant oatmeal
E	Eggs
T	Turkey (and other lean meats)
P	Peanut butter
O	Olive oil
W	Whole grains (breads and cereals)
E	Extra-protein powder (whey)
R	Raspberries (and other berries)

Adopt the Abs Diet Power 12. Eat the Abs Diet Power 12. Enjoy the Abs Diet Power 12. But, most of all, live longer and better with the Abs Diet Power 12.

HOW TO DO IT: Make sure that every meal includes at least two foods from the powerfoods list, but try to put together meals in which every food is a powerfood. The more you use the foods, the better your results. The recipes we include here will help.

GUIDELINE 3

OLD DIETS: No dessert for you!

ABS DIET: Have dessert every day!

In fact, I insist. Let's face it: There's a basic human need for sweets. In our scavenger days, our taste buds encouraged us to seek out berries and other fruits, so we'd get all the vitamins and minerals we needed. Today, we still crave sweets, and to completely eliminate them goes against human nature and guarantees only one thing—dietary failure.

So how can you fulfill your cravings for sweets but not blow a week's worth of calories on a chain-restaurant cake that's the size of an ottoman? With a powerful and sweet Abs Diet smoothie, combining as many of the powerfoods as you can—raspberries, oatmeal, peanut butter, whey powder, and milk, for instance. (See "Easy Abs Diet Smoothies" on page 18.) In each drink, you can have the taste of chocolate (whey powder comes in lots of flavors) and berries—without the guilt that typically comes from desserts. Smoothies also take up stomach space and help you avoid the blood-sugar highs and lows associated with desserts filled with simple sugars.

HOW TO DO IT: Use smoothies as snacks or replacement meals.

≫HIDDEN TREASURES

Three international foods that shouldn't be kept under wraps

Once a food is deemed healthy, it's generally well publicized. But we've found three nutritional all-stars that may have escaped your attention.

Caper berries: These grape-size fruits—harvested from a shrub found in France, Italy, and Spain—are packed with the same disease-fighting antioxidants that are in green tea and red wine. They're the mature version of the caper, so their flavor is similar but less intense. Add them to any dish in which you might find olives—such as salads, pasta, and even omelets.

Pine nuts: Harvested in Europe, Mexico, China, and the United States, these pine-tree seeds contain plenty of healthy fat and more protein per ounce than many other nuts. Their subtle, nutty taste and crunchy texture provide a perfect topping for virtually any salad, vegetable, meat, or pasta dish.

Quinoa: Although this South American seed is considered a whole grain, it's actually from the same food family as spinach and beets. And, unlike wheat and rice, it provides a healthy dose of all the essential amino acids, making it a complete protein. Another bonus: It's a good source of fiber and heart-healthy omega-3 fats. Try it as an alternative side dish to rice or pasta.

GUIDELINE 4

OLD DIETS: Count every calorie, weigh every portion, hoard points, eat meals in some sort of "zone."

ABS DIET: Have a life.

Sure, some of us really are rocket scientists. We track calories and calculate our optimum payload and energy expenditure. That's fine if it works for you. But you know what? Most of us have our hands so full with work, kids, and *CSI* reruns that we don't have time to obsess over food. So don't. Eat the Power 12, and calories and fat take care of themselves.

HOW TO DO IT: Eat meals with a balance of nutrients—making sure to include stomach satisfying high-fiber whole grains, good fats, and protein. Let your foods do the counting.

GUIDELINE 5

OLD DIETS: It's the food, stupid.

ABS DIET: It's the drink, stupid.

Your food intake can be as healthy and as disciplined as a monk's, and you can still be consuming too many calories. Between high-sugar OJ, high-fat whole milk, high-calorie sports drinks, and higher-calorie beer, it's scary how many unhealthy fats and carbohydrates we guzzle. For that reason, I want you to really examine what you drink along with and between meals.

HOW TO DO IT: Drink water, fat-free or low-fat milk, and smoothies. Coffee and tea are okay, too. But avoid whole-fat dairy products and high-sugar fruit juices. Alcohol? Best to limit yourself to two or three drinks a week, because you don't need the extra calories. And for goodness' sake, stop with the soda. Our constantly increasing soda consumption (50 gallons per person per year!) may well be the biggest reason for the obesity epidemic.

GUIDELINE 6

OLD DIETS: Don't cheat.

ABS DIET: Cheat like Jude Law at a nanny convention.

Diets used to be like marriages: If you strayed from the rules, you were done. You cheated? Forget it. Diet's over. But I want you to cheat (on the diet, that is). One meal a week, eat anything you want. Deprivation leads to resentment, which leads to a secret affair with both Ben and Jerry. But if you cut loose once a week, you'll feel in control for the other 41 meals and snacks—eating healthy will be your choice, not your chore.

HOW TO DO IT: Time your cheat meal to coincide with a party, a poker game, or your office happy hour. Just don't be surprised if, when your body adjusts to the powerfoods, you don't feel the need to cut loose. This is a diet that works with you, not against you.

Okay, now that you've had a taste of the philosophy behind the Abs Diet, let's eat. In the next pages, you'll find a day of great eating that's packed with powerfoods. Try these recipes over the next week, and you'll understand the real benefit of the Abs Diet: You don't have to choose between eating well and eating right. And a six-pack comes with every meal.

BREAKFAST OPTIONS

THE ULTIMATE POWER BREAKFAST

Powerfoods: 8

1 egg
1 cup low-fat milk
¾ cup instant oatmeal
½ cup mixed berries
1 tablespoon chopped pecans or almonds
1 teaspoon vanilla whey-protein powder
1 teaspoon ground flaxseed
½ banana, sliced
1 tablespoon plain yogurt

In a microwavable bowl, mix the egg well, then add the milk, oatmeal, berries, nuts, protein powder, and flaxseed and nuke for 2 minutes. Remove the bowl from the microwave and let the mixture cool for a minute or two. Top with the banana and yogurt.

MAKES 1 SERVING

PER SERVING: 590 CALORIES, 30 G PROTEIN, 80 G CARBOHYDRATES, 17 G FAT (4 G SATURATED), 12 G FIBER, 193 MG SODIUM

TEXAS TWO-STEP

Powerfoods: 5

1 cup cooked microwavable brown rice,
    such as Uncle Ben's
⅓ cup red beans
1 teaspoon chopped cilantro
1 egg, fried
1 tablespoon shredded low-fat Mexican-blend cheese

Mix together the microwaved rice and the beans and top with the cilantro, egg, and cheese.

MAKES 1 SERVING

PER SERVING: 379 CALORIES, 16 G PROTEIN, 55 G CARBOHYDRATES,
10 G FAT (3 G SATURATED), 7 G FIBER, 234 MG SODIUM

LUNCH OPTIONS

CRUNCH TIME

Powerfoods: 5

3 cups mixed greens
2 slices deli smoked-turkey slices, chopped
½ small Granny Smith apple, chopped
2 tablespoons grated carrot
1 tablespoon chopped pecans
1½ tablespoons Craisins (dried, sweetened cranberries)
1 tablespoon blue-cheese crumbles
1½ teaspoons olive oil
1 tablespoon balsamic vinegar

In a bowl, toss together the greens, turkey, apple, carrot, pecans, Craisins, and cheese.

In a separate bowl, combine the oil and vinegar. Pour the dressing over the salad.

MAKES 1 SERVING

PER SERVING: 296 CALORIES, 15 G PROTEIN, 31 G CARBOHYDRATES,
15 G FAT (3 G SATURATED), 7 G FIBER, 590 MG SODIUM

⟫EASY ABS DIET SMOOTHIES

EXTREME CHOCOLATE

POWERFOODS: 3

1 scoop low-fat chocolate ice cream

1 tablespoon chocolate syrup

½ cup low-fat chocolate milk

1 tablespoon chocolate whey protein powder

½ banana

3 ice cubes

Blend all ingredients.

MAKES 1 SERVING

PER SERVING: 355 CALORIES, 17 G PROTEIN, 60 G CARBS,
6 G TOTAL FAT (4 G SATURATED), 4 G FIBER, 158 MG SODIUM

DARK VADER

POWERFOODS: 4

1 scoop low-fat chocolate ice cream

½ cup reduced- fat ricotta cheese

½ cup low-fat chocolate milk

1 tablespoon chocolate whey protein powder

1 teaspoon ground flaxseed

3 ice cubes

Blend all ingredients.

MAKES 1 SERVING

PER SERVING: 400 CALORIES, 29 G PROTEIN, 40 G CARBS,
15 G TOTAL FAT (10 G SATURATED), 2 G FIBER, 315 MG SODIUM

ON A ROLL

Powerfoods: 4

¾ cup diced precooked chicken
2 tablespoons diced onion
2 tablespoons feta-cheese crumbles
1 handful romaine lettuce, chopped
1 large whole-wheat tortilla
Salsa for dipping

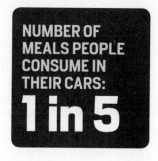

NUMBER OF MEALS PEOPLE CONSUME IN THEIR CARS: **1 in 5**

Arrange the chicken, onion, cheese, and lettuce down the center of the tortilla. Roll it tightly, then cut it in half.

Grill the roll seam-side down for 2 to 3 minutes per side, on a nonstick skillet heated to medium. Serve with salsa.

MAKES 1 SERVING

PER SERVING: 397 CALORIES, 56 G PROTEIN, 25 G CARBOHYDRATES, 10 G FAT (4 G SATURATED), 3 G FIBER, 493 MG SODIUM

PERFECT PITA

Powerfoods: 4

1 tablespoon barbecue sauce
½ cup chopped precooked chicken
1 whole-wheat pita
1 cup chopped romaine lettuce
2 tablespoons diced cucumber
1 tablespoon low-fat ranch dressing

In a microwavable dish, stir together the barbecue sauce and chicken. Microwave for 30 seconds or until hot. Stuff the chicken into each pita half.

In a bowl, toss the lettuce and cucumber with the dressing, and stuff it all into the pita.

MAKES 1 SERVING

PER SERVING: 421 CALORIES, 40 G PROTEIN, 44 G CARBOHYDRATES, 10 G FAT (2 G SATURATED), 6 G FIBER, 734 MG SODIUM

DINNER OPTIONS

SHRIMP TO NUTS

Powerfoods: 4

2 teaspoons peanut oil
¼ teaspoon red-pepper flakes
½ cup French-style green beans
⅓ cup matchstick carrots
¼ cup whole, unsalted roasted cashews
2 teaspoons reduced-sodium soy sauce
2 teaspoons orange juice
¼ teaspoon orange zest
1½ cup medium frozen shrimp, defrosted, with tails removed

Combine the oil and red pepper in a medium-hot skillet. Add the beans, carrots, cashews, soy sauce, orange juice, and orange zest and cook for 2 to 3 minutes, stirring frequently. Finally, toss in the shrimp and cook for another 2 to 3 minutes, stirring often. (Serving suggestion: Serve over brown rice.)

MAKES 2 SERVINGS

PER SERVING: 332 CALORIES, 39 G PROTEIN, 11 G CARBOHYDRATES, 15 G FAT (3 G SATURATED), 2 G FIBER, 578 MG SODIUM

BBQ-ZA

Powerfoods: 3

¼ cup barbecue sauce
1 ready-made flatbread
¼ cup canned diced tomatoes with chili peppers and onions, well drained
¾ cup precooked mesquite-flavored chicken
2 tablespoons sliced scallion
1 teaspoon diced cilantro
3 tablespoons grated, reduced-fat mozzarella cheese

Preheat the oven to 375°F. Spread the barbecue sauce on the flatbread. Top with the tomatoes, chicken, scallion, cilantro, and mozzarella. Bake for 6 minutes.

MAKES 1 SERVING

PER SERVING: 411 CALORIES, 39 G PROTEIN, 41 G CARBOHYDRATES, 10 G FAT (4 G SATURATED), 3 G FIBER, 1,059 MG SODIUM

DESSERT OPTIONS

CHOCOLATE FACTORY

Powerfoods: 4

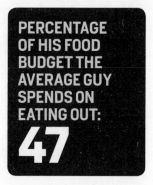

PERCENTAGE OF HIS FOOD BUDGET THE AVERAGE GUY SPENDS ON EATING OUT:
47

½ **cup** reduced-fat ricotta cheese

½ **cup** low-fat vanilla yogurt

1 teaspoon chocolate whey-protein powder

1 tablespoon chocolate syrup

1 tablespoon chopped pecans

Mix the ricotta, yogurt, protein powder, syrup, and nuts until well blended.

MAKES 1 SERVING

PER SERVING: 336 CALORIES, 20 G PROTEIN, 36 G CARBOHYDRATES, 12 G FAT (4 G SATURATED), 2 G FIBER, 209 MG SODIUM

BANANACICLES

Powerfoods: 1

4 Popsicle sticks

2 bananas, peeled and cut in half

½ **cup** chocolate sauce (the kind that forms a shell)

4 tablespoons finely chopped unsalted peanuts

Insert a Popsicle stick into the cut end of each banana piece. Pour chocolate sauce over the bananas until they're completely coated, then roll the chocolate-coated bananas in the peanuts. Freeze.

MAKES 4 SERVINGS

PER SERVING: 318 CALORIES, 4 G PROTEIN, 32 G CARBOHYDRATES, 22 G FAT (9 G SATURATED), 4 G FIBER, 21 MG SODIUM

Reprinted from *The Abs Diet 6-Minute Meals for 6-Pack Abs!* by David Zinczenko with Ted Spiker. © 2006 by Rodale Inc.

PERFECT FOODS

SLIM FAST WITH THIS DAY'S WORTH OF THE BEST MEALS AND SNACKS

BY CASSANDRA FORSYTHE

Pick a day to give this a try. Sit back and relax, we've made all of the hard decisions for you. These meals and snacks are lower in sugar and calories, but loaded with protein, fiber, and especially flavor.

BREAKFAST

7:00 A.M.: After a full 7 or 8 hours without food, your body craves a healthy dose of high-quality protein. Start your day right with at least 30 grams, along with plenty of slow-digesting carbs. Because your carbohydrate stores are low after an overnight fast, there's no better time to fill your tank. Just make sure your carbs come primarily from fruit and 100 percent whole-grain sources.

OPTION 1: STRAWBERRY-AND-BANANA WORKOUT SHAKE

If you work out first thing in the morning, choose this option, drinking half of the shake right before your session and half immediately afterward.

Blend together:

2 scoops vanilla whey-protein powder
6 ounces Yoplait Light fat-free strawberry yogurt
8 frozen strawberries
1 large banana
Plenty of ice

MAKES 1 SERVING

PER SERVING: 491 CALORIES, 52 G PROTEIN, 61 G CARBOHYDRATES, 6 G FAT (1 G SATURATED), 5 G FIBER

OPTION 2: SPICY OMELET

Make with:

1 cup Egg Beaters

1 medium egg

½ cup fresh spinach

2 mushrooms, sliced

2 tablespoons shredded light Cheddar cheese

½ cup salsa

Have on the side:

1 slice 100% whole-wheat bread with 1 tablespoon Smucker's low-sugar jelly

1 cup V8 juice

MAKES 1 SERVING

PER SERVING: 421 CALORIES, 37 G PROTEIN, 40 G CARBOHYDRATES, 11 G FAT (4 G SATURATED), 5 G FIBER

OPTION 3: PROTEIN-PACKED OATMEAL

Prepare:

1 package Nature's Path Instant Flax 'N Oats

Mix in:

1 scoop strawberry whey-protein powder
    (Choose a product that's 100% whey protein, such as Optimum Nutrition 100% Whey Gold Standard; www.optimumnutrition.com.)

3 tablespoons 1% milk

Have on the side:

1 medium pear

1 cup green tea or coffee (sweetened with Splenda)

MAKES 1 SERVING

PER SERVING: 472 CALORIES, 32 G PROTEIN, 76 G CARBOHYDRATES, 8 G FAT (1 G SATURATED), 9 G FIBER

POUNDS OF ADDED SUGAR THAT THE AVERAGE AMERICAN EATS EACH YEAR (ABOUT 23 TABLESPOONS A DAY): 74

MIDMORNING SNACK

10:00 A.M.: Eating protein- and fiber-rich meals or snacks every 2 to 3 hours helps keep your blood-sugar levels normal. This not only improves your body's ability to burn fat, but it also reduces risk factors for heart disease by lowering cholesterol and triglycerides. Frequent eating also prevents afternoon binges on useless calories, like the leftover Krispy Kremes from your morning staff meeting.

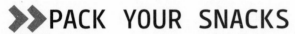PACK YOUR SNACKS

Don't leave your health at the mercy of the guy who fills the vending machine. Bring snacks with you so you'll be sure to have a healthy option.

Snacks that are 200 calories and under

Stick of string cheese (80)

Skippy brand squeeze stick of peanut butter (140)

5 cups light microwave popcorn sprinkled with hot sauce
and 1 tablespoon Romano cheese (150)

6 strawberries dipped in yogurt, drizzled with chocolate sauce (150)

Canned tuna with balsamic vinegar on whole-grain crackers (175)

1 cup reduced-sodium cottage cheese with fresh peaches and cinnamon (200)

Two handfuls of olives (200)

1 cup blackberries, blueberries, or strawberries with 6 ounces
light yogurt and 1 tablespoon low-fat granola (200)

Snacks that are 400 calories and under

One egg on a whole-grain English muffin with melted cheese (250)

Clif bar (250)

Peanut butter and jelly on a whole-grain English muffin (300)

Oatmeal with milk, brown sugar, walnuts, and any fresh or dried fruit (300)

Slice of whole-grain bread topped with peanut butter and banana (300)

$1/2$ cup hummus with roasted vegetables (400)

OPTION 1: GRAPES, CHEESE, AND HAM

1½ cups seedless grapes

2 slices fat-free American cheese singles

4 ounces Healthy Choice ham slices

MAKES 1 SERVING

PER SERVING: 352 CALORIES, 28 G PROTEIN,
51 G CARBOHYDRATES,
4 G FAT (1 G SATURATED), 2 G FIBER

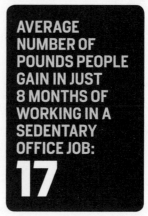

AVERAGE NUMBER OF POUNDS PEOPLE GAIN IN JUST 8 MONTHS OF WORKING IN A SEDENTARY OFFICE JOB:

17

OPTION 2: MEXI-TUNA

Mix together:

1 3-ounce can (or packet) Starkist Premium Chunk Light Tuna in Water

¾ cup canned black beans

½ cup salsa

½ cup canned green beans

MAKES 1 SERVING

PER SERVING: 335 CALORIES, 45 G PROTEIN,
41 G CARBOHYDRATES, 1 G FAT (0 G SATURATED), 15 G FIBER

OPTION 3: CHILI

Microwave:

½ can Hormel Less Sodium Chili with Beans

MAKES 1 SERVING

PER SERVING: 340 CALORIES, 18 G PROTEIN,
30 G CARBOHYDRATES, 17 G FAT (7 G SATURATED), 9 G FIBER

LUNCH

12:00 P.M.: These lunches not only are high in protein and healthy fat, but they also score low on the glycemic index. So, like the midmorning snack, they contain carbohydrates that have little impact on your blood sugar. This keeps your fat-burning furnace stoked and helps prevent the dreaded midday lull.

OPTION 1: TUNA SANDWICH

Make with:

2 slices 100% whole-wheat bread

1 3-ounce can (or packet) Starkist Premium Chunk Light Tuna in Water

1 tablespoon Hellmann's Light mayonnaise

1 tablespoon mustard

1 lettuce leaf

2 slices tomato

1 teaspoon chopped onions

1 tablespoon chopped celery

Have on the side:

1 ounce Planters mixed nuts

MAKES 1 SERVING

PER SERVING: 506 CALORIES, 45 G PROTEIN,
41 G CARBOHYDRATES, 17 G FAT (2 G SATURATED), 7 G FIBER

OPTION 2: CHEF'S SALAD

Combine:

2 cups chopped romaine lettuce

1 large hard-boiled egg

2 ounces Healthy Choice turkey breast

2 ounces Healthy Choice ham

1 ounce sliced light Cheddar cheese

1 ounce sliced light American cheese

6 cherry tomatoes

½ ounce sliced almonds

2 tablespoons Hidden Valley Original Ranch Light Dressing

(For a different flavor, try dressing your salad with olive oil and vinegar, which has 0 grams of sugar.)

MAKES 1 SERVING

PER SERVING: 493 CALORIES, 54 G PROTEIN, 20 G CARBOHYDRATES, 22 G FAT (6 G SATURATED), 4 G FIBER

MIDAFTERNOON SNACK

3:00 P.M.: As the day goes on, your ability to utilize carbohydrates for energy decreases, boosting the likelihood that they'll be stored as fat. So late afternoon is a good time to start downsizing your carb intake and increasing the amount of healthy fat you consume. This also leads to fewer total carbohydrates in your daily diet, which speeds fat loss, according to multiple studies over the past 5 years.

OPTION 1: CHEESE STICKS AND NUTS

2 sticks 2%-fat string cheese
1 ounce walnuts

MAKES 1 SERVING

PER SERVING: 307 CALORIES, 24 G PROTEIN, 5 G CARBOHYDRATES, 24 G FAT (6 G SATURATED), 2 G FIBER

OPTION 2: BEEF JERKY AND CELERY WITH PEANUT BUTTER

2 ounces beef jerky
1 celery stalk
1 tablespoon Simply Jif Creamy Peanut Butter 33% Less Sugar

MAKES 1 SERVING

PER SERVING: 277 CALORIES, 33 G PROTEIN, 14 G CARBOHYDRATES, 10 G FAT (2 G SATURATED), 3 G FIBER

OPTION 3: LOW-CARB PROTEIN BAR

1 Metabolic Drive Protein-Energy bar (www.t-nation.com) or similar product that contains fewer than 30 grams carbohydrates and 20 or more grams protein

MAKES 1 SERVING

PER SERVING: 240 CALORIES, 20 G PROTEIN, 26 G CARBOHYDRATES, 8 G FAT (3 G SATURATED), 2 G FIBER

DINNER

6:00 P.M.: Your sense of satiety, or feeling of fullness, is less sensitive in the evening than in the morning, which may help explain why you crave foods such as ice cream at night. It's also another reason it makes sense to eat a dinner that's high in protein and healthy fat, both of which keep you full longer than carbohydrates do.

OPTION 1: PANFRIED SALMON WITH BROCCOLI AND BEANS

Panfry:

1 5½-ounce salmon fillet

2 tablespoons olive oil preheated in a nonstick skillet

Panfry on medium-high heat for 4 minutes; turn and fry for another 5 minutes. Season with fresh lemon juice and dill.

Have on the side:

2 cups steamed broccoli (measured raw)

½ can dark-red kidney beans
   (Wash thoroughly, then serve without cooking.)

MAKES 1 SERVING
PER SERVING: 516 CALORIES, 56 G PROTEIN,
36 G CARBOHYDRATES, 19 G FAT (3 G SATURATED), 18 G FIBER

OPTION 2: MEAT LOAF WITH GREEN BEANS

Combine:

1 pound extra-lean ground beef

½ cup oats

½ cup Heinz OneCarb Ketchup
   (Use this version instead of regular ketchup to avoid unnecessary sugar.)

1 large egg

½ teaspoon salt

½ teaspoon pepper

2 tablespoons dried onion flakes

1 teaspoon dried mustard

1 teaspoon Worcestershire sauce

Preheat the oven to 350°F. In a baking pan, mix and form the ingredients into a loaf with your hands.

Cook for:

15 to 20 minutes.

Have on the side:

1 cup cooked green beans

MAKES 2 SERVINGS

PER SERVING: 530 CALORIES, 52 G PROTEIN,
28 G CARBOHYDRATES, 20 G FAT (9 G SATURATED), 5 G FIBER

BEFORE-BED SNACK

9:00 P.M.: Slow-absorbing proteins such as casein—the type of protein found in dairy products—deliver a steady supply of amino acids to muscle cells while you sleep, protecting your hard-earned muscle.

OPTION 1: PROTEIN PUDDING

Mix together, then chill for 1 hour:

1 scoop chocolate whey-protein powder
6 ounces 1% milk
1 teaspoon sugar-free Jell-O pudding mix

MAKES 1 SERVING

PER SERVING: 239 CALORIES, 33 G PROTEIN,
17 G CARBOHYDRATES, 4 G FAT (1 G SATURATED), 1 G FIBER

OPTION 2: COTTAGE CHEESE AND STRAWBERRIES

Mix together:

1 cup Breakstone's 2% cottage cheese
¾ cup sliced strawberries

MAKES 1 SERVING

PER SERVING: 198 CALORIES, 29 G PROTEIN,
14 G CARBOHYDRATES, 3 G FAT (0.5 G SATURATED), 3 G FIBER

HAVE AN INCREDIBLE, EDIBLE EGG

Yolking your diet could rein in your appetite. St. Louis University scientists found that people who eat eggs as part of their breakfast consume fewer calories the rest of the day than those who skip the eggs. In the study, people were given one of two breakfasts: (1) two scrambled eggs, two slices of toast, and a tablespoon of reduced-calorie fruit spread; or (2) a bagel, 2 tablespoons of cream cheese, and 3 ounces of nonfat yogurt. Even though the breakfasts were equal in calories, the egg eaters consumed 264 fewer calories by the end of the day. The researchers aren't sure why eating eggs appears to reduce hunger and food intake, but they think that the meal's higher protein and fat content may lead to greater satiety.

THINK YOUR WAY THIN

This study could cause you to lose your appetite. British researchers discovered that thinking about what you had for lunch keeps you from bingeing on afternoon snacks. During a sham taste test, scientists asked men to rate three types of salted popcorn—and encouraged them to eat as much as they wanted. Interestingly, those who were first asked to recall exactly what they'd eaten for lunch downed 30 percent less popcorn than those who were allowed to skip the review session. "Remembering recent eating might enhance awareness of how satiating the food was, which then has an effect on subsequent consumption," says study author Suzanne Higgs, PhD. Before your next afternoon snack break, take a minute to log your lunch at www.fitday.com, a free food-diary Web site.

TRY THE COOLEST DIET EVER

Researchers at the University of Illinois recently found that frozen dinners may help speed weight loss. When scientists placed two groups of men on a 1,700-calorie diet for 8 weeks, they found that those who ate one-serving packaged meals for lunch and dinner lost 45 percent more weight than men who made their own meals. "People tend to think a healthy portion is larger than it really is, which probably explains the difference between groups," says lead author Sandra Hannum, MS, RD. The biggest losers ate Uncle Ben's bowls, which typically contain 350 to 400 calories per package. Want more variety? Check product labels for frozen entrées that have a similar number of calories and at least 20 grams of protein.

QUARTER BACK

Downsizing isn't always a bad thing. Pennsylvania State University researchers discovered that by simply reducing meal portions 25 percent, people ate 10 percent fewer calories a day—without feeling any hungrier. The best place to start: Cut back on pasta and rice. An American Dietetic Association survey found that nearly 60 percent of men overestimate the serving sizes of these foods. The right answer? Half a cup of cooked pasta or rice equals one serving.

STRESS LESS

It's not your imagination: Stress really does make you crave sweets, according to researchers at Montclair State University in New Jersey. In the study, scientists provided groups of stressed and unstressed people with four bowls of different snacks: potato chips, peanuts, grapes, and M&M's. Although everyone ate the same amounts of chips and nuts, the stressed-out participants consumed five times more M&Ms and four times fewer grapes than their more laid-back counterparts. One likely reason is that foods high in simple sugar, such as candy, increase levels of serotonin, a feel-good chemical in your brain. Problem is, this may make you happier momentarily, but it won't reduce stress. Instead, manage your stress and waistline simultaneously: Danish researchers found that those who exercise at any intensity for 2 hours a week—about 17 minutes a day—are 61 percent less likely to feel highly stressed than sedentary people.

GO FISH

The next time you order spaghetti, make sure it's served *con pesce*. British scientists recently found that adding fish to pasta makes the pasta less fattening. When the researchers topped fusilli with tuna, they discovered that the glycemic index of the dish was cut in half. High-glycemic foods—such as pasta, bread, and potatoes—quickly raise your blood-sugar levels, signaling your body to store fat. "The protein in tuna helps slow the absorption of sugar into the bloodstream," says study author Helen Lightowler, PhD. Chicken, turkey, pork, and beef should have a similar effect. For a fat-fighting pasta meal you can make at home, see "Leaner Cuisines," on page 6.

More good news about fish: Swedish researchers found that men who ate fish for lunch consumed 11 percent fewer calories at dinner than those who ate beef for lunch. Interestingly, both meals contained the same amounts of calories, protein, fat, and carbohydrates. "The protein in fish takes longer to digest than that found in beef and chicken," says lead study author Stephan Rössner, PhD. "So eating fish may help you feel full longer and may reduce your appetite at your next meal."

PERCENTAGE OF MEN TRYING TO LOSE WEIGHT WHO EXERCISE BUT DON'T CHANGE THEIR DIETS:

61

PUT DOWN THAT TV DINNER

University of Massachusetts scientists found that people who watch TV during a meal consume, on average, 288 more calories than those who don't chew while changing channels. In the study, researchers had groups of people eat pizza or macaroni and cheese while either watching *Seinfeld* or listening to music. When intakes were tallied, the scientists determined that the television viewers downed 36 percent more calories from the pizza and 71 percent more from the mac and cheese. "When you're distracted by a TV show, your brain may not recognize that you're full as fast," says study author Elliott Blass, PhD.

GET MOOOO-VING

Until now, the weight-loss benefits of dairy have been measured only in total pounds. But a new study of 827 men and women found that daily consumption of three or more servings of dairy foods seems to target belly fat. In fact, the people with the highest intakes had the leanest midsections—by an average of nearly 2 inches. The reason? The calcium that accompanies dairy foods may block fat absorption and make fat less likely to be stored in the abdominal region, speculates lead researcher Fereidoun Azizi, MD. It's easy to join the calcium club: Drink a glass of milk with breakfast, eat a slice of cheese with your lunch, and have a cup of yogurt for an afternoon snack.

GET OUT OF CANDY LAND

Forget the glass ceiling in the office; we're worried about the glass candy bowl. A Cornell University study reveals that people ate twice as many Hershey's Kisses from a clear office candy bowl as from one that was opaque. The workers also gobbled more when either bowl was less than 6 feet from their desks.

HAVE ONE ON US

Regularly drinking small amounts of alcohol may help deflate a beer belly. In a recent study of 8,000 people, Texas Tech University researchers determined that those who downed a daily drink were 54 percent less likely to have a weight problem than teetotalers. Two drinks a day resulted in a 41 percent risk reduction. But that's where the trend ends. Consumption of three or more daily drinks increases your risk of obesity, says study author Ahmed A. Arif, MD, PhD. The scientists aren't sure why moderate alcohol intake has a gut-busting effect, but they point out that it appears any type of drink will work, as long as you stick to these amounts for each serving: 12 ounces of beer, 4 ounces of wine, or 1 ounce of liquor.

THE PERFECT DIET

A simple test that measures insulin may soon help predict what type of diet will work best for you. Researchers at Tufts University found that people who naturally secreted the highest levels of insulin—a hormone that signals your body to store fat—lost more weight on a low-sugar diet than on one that allowed all types of carbohydrates. (Both diets contained the same number of calories.) Those with normal insulin function fared just as well with either approach.

TINY HELPERS

Scientists at Utah State University are conducting experiments with nanoparticles to see if the super-tiny medical devices could connect with fat receptors in the small intestine. In theory, this might trick the body into feeling fuller on less food.

EFFORTLESS WEIGHT LOSS

Satisfying your sugar craving may actually help you shed unwanted pounds. A "sweet" fiber known as oligofructose has been shown to help men lose weight effortlessly. Belgian scientists recently noted that people who consumed just 1½ teaspoons of the nutrient twice a day ate 5 percent fewer total calories. For the average guy, that could add up to a 13-pound loss in a year. Try Sweet Perfection (www.lowcarbspecialties. com) in your coffee or tea. It's a sugar substitute made from more than 90 percent oligofructose; 1½ teaspoons contains almost 5 grams of fiber and only one-third the calories of table sugar.

THE SUSHI DIET

Weight-loss kelp is on the way. Japanese scientists found that a compound in brown seaweed targets belly fat. When researchers injected rats with fucoxanthin, the rodents lost up to 10 percent of their body weight, primarily from their midsections. Why? Fucoxanthin appears to stimulate UCP1, a protein that causes abdominal fat to break down. Humans can't get enough fucoxanthin to experience the benefits simply by eating seaweed, but the researchers hope to use the compound to develop an anti-obesity supplement in 3 to 5 years.

AERO GARDENS

Long winters shouldn't stifle your supply of fresh produce. This high-tech indoor-gardening system pumps out vegetables at five times the speed of plain old dirt, and no *E. coli*! It mists exposed roots with a nutrient-rich haze and carefully schedules their light exposure with an overhead LED lamp. Call it hippie hydroponics. But as goofy as an indoor garden seems, it really works. We went from seeds to salad in 2 months with the arugula kit. Tomatoes, chili peppers, and herbs are available as well. $150. www.aerogrow.com

LOSE YOUR GUT

5 WAYS TO SET GOALS THAT GET RESULTS

1. **SET THREE GOALS.** Make an optimal goal, a fairly ambitious goal, and a minimum goal. This will give you some latitude in defining success. "Men want to think that everything will go along as planned," says Martin Binks, PhD, director of behavioral health at the Duke Diet and Fitness Center. "By giving yourself several options, you'll always be on track, even if you've only reached the minimum."

2. **STOP THINKING** you have to slim down overnight. Instead, set incremental goals, such as trying to lose a pound this week, which will lead you to change your habits. At the end of the week, reset. Always keep your goals right in front of you, and measure them in days or even weeks.

3. **IGNORE "BEFORE" AND "AFTER"** advertisements common in most bodybuilding magazines. This won't come as a shocker, but a study in the journal *Eating and Weight Disorders* found that these comparison ads raise unrealistic expectations.

4. **DON'T FOCUS EXCLUSIVELY** on one goal, including a diet. "There needs to be time when you're not the person who is trying to lose weight; when you're just a guy," says Dr. Binks. Have a life.

5. **LOSE JUST 5 TO 10 PERCENT** of your body weight. According to researchers at the Mayo Clinic, this can eliminate the need for high-blood-pressure meds, cut your diabetes risk by 58 percent, reduce your heart-disease risk by 4 percent, and lower your odds of having sleep apnea.

If a pound is 3,500 calories and I cut 7,000 calories a week, I should lose 2 pounds per week, right?

If it were that easy, we wouldn't be subjected to *Celebrity Fit Club*. If you cut 7,000 calories in a week, don't expect to feel 2 pounds lighter. The reason? You have to fuel your body for weight loss. If you just cut calories, your body compensates by lowering its energy use, says Keith Berkowitz, MD, of the Center for Balanced Health in New York City.

Instead, increase the rate at which your body burns fat by replacing starchy carbs with good fats, fiber, and protein. Carbs keep insulin levels high, says Dr. Berkowitz. "And the more insulin, the more fat your body will make." So, sure, cut those calories—1,000 calories roughly equals a bagel with cream cheese, a grande mocha, and a 16-ounce soda. Then speed your fat burn by eating 8 to 10 ounces of protein (chicken, beef, or fish) and 4 to 5 cups of high-fiber vegetables or fruit a day. Spice up your breakfast of eggs and fruit with vegetables. Exercise, and after a couple of months, you'll see your weight loss average out to 2 pounds a week, says Dr. Berkowitz.

I always gorge myself when I'm at a buffet. How can I stop?

Avoid too much variety. I know that's tough at a buffet. But the more varied the foods, the more you'll fool your body's fullness detectors. That's the idea behind *The Flavor Point Diet*, by David Katz, MD, a member of *Men's Health*'s advisory board. When you cycle through sugary condiments, salty fried foods, and savory meats, each new flavor turbocharges your appetite. Even worse, loading up on flavors desensitizes you to each one, so you need to eat more to get your fix. Cut down on the sweet stuff where it doesn't belong and that Chocolate Volcano will be easier to resist.

What's the worst trap of holiday eating?

This idea of a holiday season. The people who pack on winter pounds cut loose for the entire month between Thanksgiving and Christmas. Look at it as three separate holidays—including New Year's—and splurge on those 3 days. If you must, allow yourself two small indulgences a day—a chocolate at work, an Irish coffee at a party.

What are the healthiest choices on a Chinese take-out menu?

Look for foods you can recognize. "The biggest red flags are dishes in which you can't tell what the meat is because it's breaded and fried or covered in glop," says Bonnie Taub-Dix, RD, an American Dietetic Association spokeswoman and nutritionist in New York City. That disqualifies dishes like General Tso's chicken (apologies, sir!) and sweet-and-sour everything. Anything steamed is healthy, but favor chicken, shrimp, or pork. "Most beef dishes are made with heavier, fattier sauces." White sauces are generally better than dark, but consider black-bean sauce for the added protein and nutrients. Finally, eat Chinese-style: a little of this, a little of that, lots of vegetables, spread out over a long time. Your stomach will let you know you've had enough before you've scarfed down an entire carton.

SAUCES: Order the sauce on the side. You won't put on as much as they will, so you'll cut your fat and sodium intakes.

NOODLES: Noodle dishes are never a healthy alternative. They're made with lots of oil to keep the strands from sticking.

FRIED RICE: Don't confuse fried rice with healthier brown rice. Fried rice is just white rice that's turned brown from soy sauce and oil. It's high in sodium and fat.

MYSTERY MEAT: If you can't recognize the meat, it means there's too much fat-soaked breading on it. Best bet: steamed entrees.

FORTUNE COOKIE: It's nutritionally harmless. In fact, skip the table noodles—which are as healthful as french fries—and ask for the cookie early if you need to nibble.

SOY SAUCE: Ask if they have low-sodium soy. Each tablespoon of the regular stuff has up to four times the recommended daily allowance of salt.

Some restaurants do small-plate menus. Is that supposed to help me lose weight?

According to new research, we suffer from "unit bias," which means we tend to be satisfied based on what's served to us, regardless of portion size. Take advantage and start small: One or two small plates per person may do the same to satisfy body and brain as that 18-ounce T-bone.

What's the best bread for weight loss?

The bread aisle isn't as visually stimulating as a sorority house, but it has as many choices. Slice away calories with thin-sliced bread. (On bread labels, one serving equals one slice, so double the numbers for a sandwich.) Include fiber in your search. "Three to 5 grams per serving is good," says Lola O'Rourke, a spokeswoman for the American Dietetic Association. To find healthier breads, look for the Whole Grains Council's new labeling system, adopted by many big bakers: A "Good Source" stamp means a half serving of whole grains per slice; "Excellent Source" means a full serving; "100 percent Excellent Source" means a full serving with no refined grains.

My girlfriend wants me to go vegetarian. Will I lose weight?

Sure—just don't pig out on chocolate raisins, pastries, and cheese fries. A healthy vegetarian diet includes high-fiber, low-calorie-density foods (beans, broccoli) that make you feel fuller faster. You might consider a partially vegetarian diet including low-fat dairy, fish, and eggs to maintain protein intake without packing on saturated fat and calories.

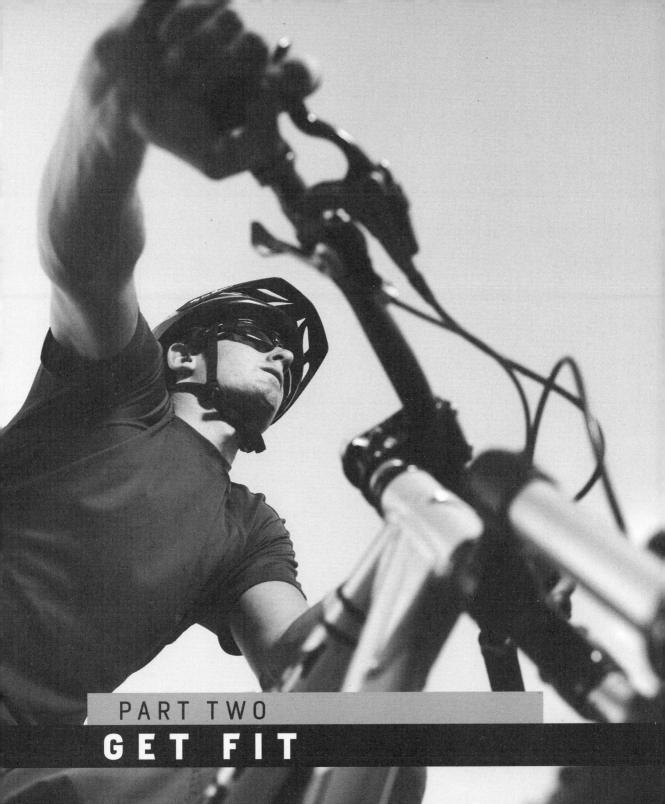

PART TWO
GET FIT

THE STATUTES OF STRETCHING

SO YOU THINK YOU KNOW HOW TO STRETCH? GUESS
AGAIN. USE THIS MYTH-BUSTING PLAN FOR
BREAKTHROUGHS IN FLEXIBILITY, PERFORMANCE,
AND INJURY PREVENTION

BY BILL HARTMAN, PT, CSCS

Unless you need to build your tolerance for boredom, most stretching is
a waste of time. After all, when you review the research, it's clear that
the most widely held principles of flexibility training simply don't work.
Which is why few guys ever stick with it and even regular practitioners
struggle to touch their toes. Worse, follow those age-old rules closely,
and studies show that you'll actually be more likely to suffer a pulled
muscle than if you hadn't stretched at all.

   That's why it's time we rewrite the book on stretching and provide
you with a flexibility plan that's not only effective, but also simple, fast,
and painless. Your first order of business is to forget everything your
high-school gym coach, workout partner, or yoga-loving girlfriend ever
told you about stretching. Then memorize the new rules that follow. The
benefit? You'll reduce your risk of injuries, improve your overall athleticism, and have an easier time tying your shoes.

FLEXIBILITY 101

Before we get to the rules, it's important to understand the basic—but typically misunderstood—science of stretching. First, a couple of definitions. There are two major types of stretching: static and dynamic.

You're probably more familiar with the former. For instance, a static stretch for your hamstrings is what you think it is—a movement in which you lean forward until you feel a slight discomfort in the target muscle, and then stretch the muscle by holding that position for a few seconds.

Although it's often prescribed as an injury-prevention measure, static stretching before a workout might be the worst of all strategies. Because it forces the target muscle to relax, it temporarily makes it weaker. As a

▶▶FROM MEAT TO MUSCLE

Here's how steak makes you grow.

1. Breaking down the meat: The process starts in your mouth with the mechanical digestion of food: Your teeth cut, tear, and mash the steak into smaller particles, mixing it with saliva to form a semisolid lump.

2. Digesting the protein: Once swallowed, the pulverized beef moves down your esophagus and lands in your stomach. Here, enzymes such as pepsin chemically break the steak into strands of amino acids. The whole mess is now more of a liquid called chyme.

3. Creating usable parts: From your stomach, the chyme passes into your small intestines. Here, additional enzymes—trypsin and chymotrypsin—act on the amino acid strands to break them into even smaller parts, until only single and double amino acids remain.

4. Preparing for delivery: The amino acids are then transported through the cells that line the walls of your intestines and into your bloodstream, a process called absorption. They're now ready to be sent to your muscles via your blood vessels.

5. Building the muscle: Once they reach your muscles, amino acids are delivered to the cells by way of capillaries. There, the amino acids help repair damaged fibers. In fact, muscle-protein synthesis can't occur unless amino acids are readily available—all the more reason to eat some protein at every meal.

result, a strength imbalance can occur between opposing muscle groups. For example, stretching your hamstrings causes them to become significantly weaker than your quadriceps. And that may make you more susceptible to muscle strains, pulls, and tears in the short term.

PERCENTAGE OF MEN WHO WANT DEFINED ABS MORE THAN ANY OTHER PHYSICAL CHARACTERISTIC:

53

Static stretching also reduces bloodflow to your muscles and decreases the activity of your central nervous system—meaning it inhibits your brain's ability to communicate with your muscles, which limits your capacity to generate force. The bottom line: Never perform static stretching before you work out or play sports.

Now, before you abandon static stretching for good, realize that it does have value. That's because improving your "passive" flexibility through static stretches is beneficial in the nonathletic endeavors of everyday life—such as bending, kneeling, and squatting. All you have to know is the right stretch for the right time.

THE RULES OF STATIC STRETCHING

WHEN: Any time of day, except before a workout

WHY: To improve general flexibility

HOW: Apply these guidelines:

Stretch twice a day, every day. Any less frequently and you won't maintain your gains in flexibility—which is why most flexibility plans don't work. Twice a day may seem like a lot, but each "session" will require as little as 4 minutes of your time. Also, there's no need to "warm" your muscles before stretching; that's a myth. So you can stretch at work, while you're watching TV, or while you're grilling burgers.

Keep in mind that duration matters. You can increase passive flexibility with a static stretch that's held for as little as 5 seconds, but you get optimal gains by holding it between 15 and 30 seconds, the point of diminishing returns.

Finally, do just one stretch for each tight muscle. Because most of the improvements in flexibility are made on the first stretch, repeating the same movement provides little benefit.

WHAT: Use these movements to stretch your entire body. Do for all but number 2, switch sides and repeat the stretch with the opposite arm or leg.

1. **UPPER TRAPEZIUS:** Place your left hand on your head and position your right arm behind your back. Gently pull your head toward your shoulder.

2. **LATISSIMUS DORSI:** Kneel on the floor so your quads are perpendicular with the floor. Keeping your back straight and parallel to the floor, rest your wrists on a Swiss ball. Then push your arms into the Swiss ball and your chest toward the floor.

⟫THE MINIMALIST WORKOUT

Get big results in almost no time

Use this 3-day total-body workout, designed by Alwyn Cosgrove, CSCS, to muscle up in less than 90 minutes a week. By incorporating the laws of functional anatomy, it works every muscle in your body with just five exercises. Building brawn has never been faster—or simpler.

How to do it: Perform this workout 3 days a week, resting a day after each session.

Do the same exercises each workout, but vary the sets, repetitions, and rest periods according to the chart below. (One exception: For the Swiss-ball pike, do 12 to 15 repetitions every session.)

For the first exercise (1), use straight sets, so that you complete all sets of the movement before moving on to the next.

Then perform each subsequent pair of exercises (2A and 2B, 3A and 3B) as alternating sets, resting for the prescribed amount of time after each. So you'll complete 1 set of exercise 2A, rest, do 1 set of exercise 2B, rest, and repeat. After you've finished all sets of both exercises, move on to the other pair.

1. Wide-grip deadlift: Set a barbell on the floor and stand facing it. Squat down and grab it with an overhand grip that's twice shoulder width. With your back flat and head up, stand up with the barbell, pulling your shoulder blades back. Slowly lower the

3. **CALVES:** Stand in front of a wall with your right leg slightly bent and your left leg straight and your left foot on the ground a few feet behind your right. Place your hands on the wall at eye level and lean forward to stretch.

4. **QUADRICEPS:** Kneel in front of a sturdy box or bench. Place your left foot on the floor with your knee bent at a 90-degree angle. With your right knee bent and on the floor, place the toes of your right foot on the bench. Push your hips forward while keeping your torso upright.

5. **PECTORALS:** Stand next to a wall, with your right shoulder toward the wall. Bend your right arm so your elbow is at a 90-degree angle.

---

bar to the starting position.

    2A. Dumbbell incline press: Lie on your back on a bench that's set to a low incline and hold a pair of dumbbells at the sides of your chest. Press the dumbbells up and together. Pause, then lower the weights back to the starting position.

    2B. Cable row: Attach a straight bar to the cable and position yourself in a cable-row machine. Grab the bar with an overhand, shoulder-width grip. Without moving your torso, pull the bar to your abdomen. Pause, then slowly return to the starting position.

    3A. Wide-grip lat pulldown: Grab the bar with an overhand grip that's about twice shoulder width and sit up straight. Without moving your torso, pull the bar down to your chest. Pause, then slowly return to the starting position.

    3B. Swiss-ball pike: Get into pushup position, but instead of placing your feet on the floor, rest your shins on a Swiss ball. Raise your hips as high as you can as you roll the ball toward your body. Pause, then return to the start by lowering your hips and rolling the ball backward.

    For each exercise, take 3 seconds to lower the weight, pause for 1 second, then take 1 second to lift it.

Workout	Sets	Reps	Rest
Monday	4	5	90 seconds
Wednesday	2	15	30 seconds

Place your hand, wrist, and forearm against the wall, then move your shoulder forward.

6. **HAMSTRINGS:** Stand a few feet away from a sturdy box or bench, facing the bench. Place your hands on your hips. With your left foot on the floor, place your right foot on the box or bench, then lean forward from the hips until you feel a stretch.

A dynamic stretch is the opposite of a static stretch. In this version, you quickly move a muscle in and out of a stretched position. Example: A body-weight lunge is a dynamic stretch for your quadriceps and hips.

Improvements in flexibility are specific to your body position and speed of movement. So if you do only static stretching, you'll primarily boost your flexibility in that exact posture while moving at a slow speed. This has limited carryover to the flexibility you need in sports and weight training, which require your muscles to stretch at fast speeds in various body positions. Dynamic stretching is necessary because it improves your "active" flexibility, the kind you need in every type of athletic endeavor.

Dynamic stretching also excites your central nervous system, and increases bloodflow, and strength and power production. So it's the ideal warmup for any activity. And when you regularly perform both dynamic and static stretches, some of the flexibility improvements from one will transfer to the other.

THE RULES OF DYNAMIC STRETCHING

WHEN: As a warmup before any type of workout or sport

WHY: To improve performance and reduce injury risk

HOW: Perform five to eight body-weight exercises or calisthenics at a slow tempo and in a comfortable range of motion. Increase your range and speed with each repetition, until you're performing the movement quickly from start to finish. Do 1 set of 10 repetitions of each exercise, one after the other.

WHAT: Try this sample routine of movements that are probably already familiar to you: jumping jacks, arm circles, trunk rotations, front lunges, side lunges, high knees, and body-weight squats. (If you need instructions, go to www.menshealth.com/stretching.)

YOUR INNER TRIATHLETE

THINK YOU CAN'T RUN A TRIATHLON?
YES, YOU CAN! USE THIS PLAN TO GET
FASTER, FITTER, AND STRONGER THAN EVER

BY BILL STIEG

The harbor seal let me know that everything was going to be okay. It didn't say (or bark) anything, though we were certainly close enough for conversation, bobbing a few strokes apart in the swells beyond the breakers off Zuma Beach in Malibu.

The seal was sleek, serene, and floating comfortably. So was I. It was at that moment that I realized, serenely, that the triathlon the next day would be no problem. I might struggle on the bike and shuffle through the run, but I'd survive the swim. This had been a concern. But I learned during this 20-minute practice swim that in a wetsuit, in salt water, you don't sink. Just like a seal.

That was the 174th surprise for me and my five *Men's Health* teammates, triathlon virgins all, in the 3 months since we'd begun training for the Nautica Malibu Triathlon. Giddy buoyancy among sea mammals ranked up there with surprises like "Man, bikes are expensive!" and "This Body-Glide gives me an idea." But the overarching realization was "Anyone can do this."

We were living (and swimming, biking, running) proof. Six men of varying ages, body types, and fitness levels, active but not insanely so, easily finished our "sprint" triathlon—a half-mile swim, 18-mile bike ride, and 4-mile run. An Ironman this was not. That's a 2.4-mile swim, 112-mile ride, and full 26.2-mile marathon. That's insane.

But in everyday conversation, nobody hears the distances. They hear only "triathlon." The work-to-reward ratio was ideal. The post-event soreness, less than after a 10-mile run. The afterglow, sublime. We're all doing it again this year.

Nothing should stop you, either. "The biggest misconception about tri-athlons is that training for them has to encompass your life," says Cameron Widoff, the top American in last year's Ironman World Championship. "The key is getting over that fear of what it takes to do one. The fear is baseless most of the time. And doing a sprint makes the most sense."

So find your apprehensions below, learn from our experience, then sign up for a sprint triathlon and commence training. In 2 months, you'll be ready for the starting line.

SWIMMING

THE WORRIES: Your swimming stroke is thrash-and-sink, with an occa-sional grab-the-side. You haven't swum more than a length since high school. In fact, you're pretty sure you hate swimming. It's cold and wet and boring.

THE SURPRISE: We love swimming. Four of our six team members were pathetic swimmers at the outset. But each of us learned that taking just a few lessons (in person or from a book or DVD) leads to quick, steep improvement. Concentrating on technique makes laps intriguing—that one felt fast; what did I do differently? And as a workout, swimming rules supreme: a lung-expanding, upper-body-building, big-breakfast-justifying calorie incinerator that leaves no sore joints afterward. We all benefited from the insights of Terry Laughlin, a swimming wizard in the Catskills who sells his wisdom via his Web site, www.totalim-mersion.net. The easiest approach is to buy his books or DVDs, or, bet-ter yet, take a TI (Total Immersion) swimming workshop.

THE TRAINING: Most of us hit the water two or three times a week, progressing in about 12 weeks from a couple of gasping laps to a work-out that lasted 30 to 60 minutes and covered half a mile to a mile. Here's what we learned along the way.

When swimming, focus on balance. Most beginners hold their torsos and heads up, doglike. This creates poor balance and makes your lower body sink—forcing your muscles to work hard to keep you horizontal, says Laughlin. When you let your heavy head hang down with your chest, your legs will rise, allowing you to glide through the water with far less effort.

>>TRIATHLON GEAR, SIMPLIFIED

First-timers don't need much equipment and can borrow most of it. But here are the essentials, along with upgrades to consider if you plan to stick with it for the long haul.

THE SWIM

Need: Goggles, quick-wicking tri shorts, and a tri top or lightweight running shirt; a wetsuit if it's an ocean swim

Regular bike shorts absorb too much water. Stay comfortable in an outfit like the Zoot Trifit Racesuit, which wicks moisture and dries quickly. ($95. www.zootsports.com)

Upgrade: A sleeveless wetsuit like the Xterra Ventilator feels like cheating, but it isn't. ($190. www.xterrawetsuits.com)

Fantasy: The new Orca Apex is thin and slippery smooth, but it contains hidden air pockets for more buoyancy. ($550. www.orca.com)

THE RIDE

Need: Any tuned bike, plus socks and a helmet

Use your old road bike (get it tuned up) or borrow one—or buy a nice, affordable new one like the Jamis Ventura Comp ($980, www.jamisbikes.com). Even a mountain bike with slick tires will get you through a sprint.

Upgrade: A tri bike's upright seat tube and handlebar extensions called aero bars will make you more aerodynamic—crucial in a race in which drafting isn't allowed. Consider the Kuota K-Factor. ($2,600 and up. www.all3sports.com)

Fantasy: A one-piece carbon-frame bike like the Cervélo P3 Carbon lasts forever and absorbs road vibration like magic. ($4,500. www.cervelo.com)

THE RUN

Need: A pair of broken-in running shoes

Upgrade: Need a new pair? Try the New Balance 825, highly rated by *Runner's World* magazine, with stickier rubber on the forefoot for better traction. Make sure you've trained in them for at least a month. ($90. www.newbalance.com)

Fantasy: Monitoring your heart rate is the surest way to guarantee you're not overdoing your training. The Garmin Forerunner 305 is a watch-size wonder. ($375. www.garmin.com)

To take a breath, roll your entire body. That means your head stays in the water, but your face rotates with your torso so you can breathe. This ensures that you don't lose momentum each time you come up for air, says Laughlin.

Pierce the water, don't try to overcome it. Make your body as long and narrow as possible by extending an arm and slipping your hand cleanly into the water "as if through a mail slot." Laughlin says this eliminates much of the thrashing that slows guys down.

If you'll be wearing a wetsuit in the race, be sure to practice in it. "It feels different than free swimming," says triathlon coach Mark Allen, a six-time Ironman winner. Do a few 100s in the pool with and without it so you have the confidence that it's going to make you faster, even though it feels slower.

Relax. "There's no limitation on strokes," says Joe Friel, author of *Your First Triathlon*. You can grab safety boats and surfboards and buoys for a rest. In my race, I switched from the crawl to the breaststroke, the sidestroke, even the elementary backstroke, and never got tired. (And still beat a few guys in my age group out of the water.)

BIKING

THE WORRIES: You haven't ridden a bike for a long distance since you were 15 and awaiting your driver's license. You don't own a road bike. You hate training, because it seems every car is trying to run you off the road.

THE SURPRISE: Fast is fun. If you're primarily a runner, prepare to become addicted to speed and fresh air. This is a workout that you'll adjust schedules for, and haul your bike across the county to find clear roads for.

THE TRAINING: We did a couple of bike rides a week, though we wanted to do more. We'd average 15 to 16 miles per hour, with a typical ride lasting about an hour, longer on weekends. What we learned:

Match your practice course to your race course. If the race is going to be hilly, find some hills. Same with long flat stretches, which can seem harder than hills because of monotony and headwinds.

Stay out of high gear. "You want your legs spinning the entire time," says Rachel Cosgrove, CSCS, a triathlon coach in Santa Clarita, Cali-

▶▶8 WEEKS TO RACE DAY

This plan from Rachel Cosgrove, CSCS, will get you in sprint-triathlon shape in 3 hours a week. Numbers indicate minutes, at a challenging pace. For more, see www.menshealth.com/8weekplan.

DAY	Week 1	Week 2	Week 3	Week 4	Week 5	Week 6	Week 7	Week 8
MONDAY	Swim: 20	Off	Off	Off	Off	Off	Off	Off
TUESDAY	Off	Swim: 30	Swim: 30	Swim: 30	Swim: 800 meters	Swim: 1000 meters	Swim: 1000 meters	Cycle: 30
WEDNESDAY	Run: 20	Run: 25	Run: 30	Run: 30	Cycle: 45	Cycle: 60	Run: 4 miles	Swim: 500 meters
THURSDAY	Off	Off	Off	Off	Off	Off	Off	Off
FRIDAY	Swim: 20	Swim: 30	Swim: 30	Run: 20	Run: 3 miles	Run: 4 miles	Swim: 1000 meters	Off
SATURDAY	Run: 20	Cycle: 45	Cycle: 45 Run: 10	Cycle: 20	Swim: 20	Swim: open water	Cycle: 24 miles	Travel to race
SUNDAY	Cycle: 30	Run: 25	Cycle: 60	Cycle: 20 miles	Cycle: 12 miles	Cycle 15 miles Run: 2 miles	Run: 3 miles	Race Day!

fornia. Use a gear high enough to allow you to pedal without coasting for the duration of your workout. This will reduce fatigue in your muscles, compared with using lower gears, in which you have to exert more force. Also, make sure you pedal in full circles, pulling one pedal as you push the other.

Practice transitioning from a swim to a bike ride. It's not as jarring as the bike-to-run transition (or T2, as we veteran triathletes call it),

PERCENTAGE OF MEN AGES 45 TO 54 WHO EXERCISE REGULARLY:

33

but you at least need to practice pulling that wetsuit off and stepping into your bike shoes. A couple of times should do it.

When you race, go into a lower gear in the last quarter mile or so and stretch. Friel's approach: "Stand up on the pedals and drop your heel to stretch your calf. For your hamstrings, lean forward. Do this on both sides. Standing up straight and pushing your hips forward will help stretch your back." You'll decrease the odds of cramping as you run.

During an event, use the bike ride to take in liquids, gels, or an energy bar (though these last two aren't necessary in a sprint). "It's more efficient, and it sets you up for the run," Widoff says.

RUNNING

THE WORRIES: Running hurts your knees. You struggle to run 3 miles on a normal day, let alone at the end of 90 minutes of effort.

THE SURPRISE: You'll become a better runner by running less. Swimming and biking help your legs recover from the pounding of running. Come the last leg, you're closer to exhilaration than exhaustion. You didn't drown, you didn't crash. You're on solid ground, and your feet are moving. You'll finish.

THE TRAINING: For most men, this part of training gets short shrift, but it doesn't matter. For the creaky-kneed, swimming and biking will feel great. Regular runners—the biggest contingent of beginner triathletes—will find the shortish distances (3 or 4 miles, or 10 kilometers) no problem. Here's how to ensure peak performance.

Concentrate on improving your turnover, or cadence. Faster runners' feet spend little time on the pavement and strike the ground about 90 times a minute (per foot), Allen says. Regular folks' cadences are in the 70s. To adjust yours, shorten your stride so you take faster, more frequent steps.

Practice several times dismounting from the bike and running. "It's a unique experience—your legs feel like rubber," says Friel, though mine felt more like stumps. "You're training your body for that weirdness and cramping that can happen," says Widoff. Allen didn't start winning the Ironman until he began doing these "brick" workouts—teaching his body to adjust.

Swing your arms forward, like a sprinter. Most men allow their arms to move across their body when they run long distances, reducing their efficiency. The trick is to "pretend you're holding ice-cream cones," says Cosgrove. "This keeps all your momentum moving straight ahead and requires you to expend less energy." And that means you'll be able to run faster and with less effort.

In pacing yourself, "pay close attention to your breathing and forget your legs," says Friel. "Breathing is a better indicator of how hard you're running. Your legs will always tell you if you're going too slowly." The best gauge? If you're breathing too hard to talk in short spurts of three or four words at a time, you aren't going to last long.

Do nothing new on race day, says Cosgrove. Wear the same shorts you trained in, don't don a new pair of shoes, and consume the same sports drink or juice that you're used to. Even small changes could cause chafing, blisters, or stomach problems.

≫ THE ANATOMY OF MUSCLE

Here's a microscopic view of your muscles.

Muscle fiber: A single muscle cell, which contains several hundred to several thousand myofibrils

Sarcoplasm: A semifluid membrane that surrounds the myofibril and contains structures—such as mitochondria—that provide energy for muscular contraction

Fascicle: A bundle of several muscle fibers

Capillaries: Tiny blood vessels that deliver nutrients and enzymes to the muscle fibers

Muscle: A bundle of fascicles that are enclosed in a sheath of connective tissue called fascia

Myofibril: A collection of thousands of tiny proteins that together generate force to help a cell contract

Tendon: Tough connective tissue that attaches muscle to bone

MOVIE MAKEOVERS

USE SOME SILVER-SCREEN MOTIVATION TO SCULPT A STAR-QUALITY BODY

BY MIKEL JOLLETT

You can find the motivation to get in shape in the oddest of places.

Some guys find it in a doctor's office after a sobering chest exam or blood test or biopsy. Others find it at a high-school reunion when That Girl from 10th-grade biology doesn't recognize them through the haze of cheap vodka, male-pattern baldness, and so many forgotten years. As any good Russian novelist could tell you, life reaches a crossroads—and big changes follow—when sex seems less likely than death.

I found my motivation in the back of a movie theater in Santa Monica, California. That's where Brad Pitt comes in, but more about him later.

I was 25 years old, working a hundred hours a week in an office. I hadn't really set out for that life, but you know how those things go. You'd trade a kidney for an extra zero at the end of your paycheck, and so on. My days were filled with 5-year plans, capital-amortization reports, key-performance indices—i.e., the tortured lexicon of the modern office. For the first time in my life, there wasn't much time for exercise. Hell, there wasn't much time for anything but sleep and work. And eating.

Why do so many office events involve food? The candy jar on the secretary's desk. Doughnuts at morning budget meetings. Rubbery chicken lunches at the Yale Club. Steak dinners with board members. It's like we're trying to feed some existential hunger, trying to fill a dark void at the center of office life with caramels, Hershey's Kisses, and muffin baskets. People eat at the office for the same reason they drink at a bar: to forget they're there.

I don't know exactly when it got away from me. In college, on the track team, I had been all–Pac 10 in the 10,000 meters, a svelte 148 pounds whipping around the oval at 70 seconds per quarter mile. At that age, those of us on the cross-country team, those of us who ran 12 to 15 miles a day and ate mountains of food at night, felt like wild beasts. Like we were born to leap boulders, like we were panting, pawing, screaming to run. It's probably mixed up with some milk-tooth adolescent fantasy, but we really felt like we were pushing the limits of mortality. All that pain and strain and exhaustion and exhilaration.

PERCENTAGE OF MEN WHO'VE GONE 2 OR MORE MONTHS WITHOUT WORKING OUT: 54

How far can we go? How fast can we run? How much can we take? Let's find out.

But by age 25, after 3 years in office purgatory, 3 years of meetings and dinners and lunches and drinks, I was up to 225 pounds. Sitting there, listening to these middle-aged men make jokes about their wives over two-martini lunches, I felt caged, fenced in, trapped, old, tired, bored, fat.

I would find myself walking the fluorescent-lit corridors of that ungodly building with reams of green-and-white printout paper covered with endless rows of numbers, a big, round gut hanging over the 38-inch waistline of my green slacks, seething about the budget. "Have you seen these numbers, people?" Every now and then, I'd catch a glimpse of my reflection in the office glass and wonder who the fat man was.

Then it happened. In that movie theater in Santa Monica. *Fight Club.* I know that sounds trite. I know it should have been the birth of my first child or something. But it was *Fight Club* that did it. I remember seeing Marla Singer (played by Helena Bonham Carter), with that ragged eyeliner and waifish body. She was just so trashy and dirty and hot and broke. And Tyler Durden (Brad Pitt) lived in this abandoned house in the middle of nowhere with the anonymous narrator (Ed Norton). All they ever did was get in fights, wreak havoc, work out, and make fun of office automatons. Though it all ended miserably—but triumphantly!—with that Pixies song when those buildings blew up, God, my life just seemed so tame by comparison, so forgettable, so compliant. I thought, What the hell am I doing? I'm 25 years old.

I saw the movie four times in 1 week. And I cracked. I quit my job. I dumped my girlfriend. I started working out constantly. Running, swimming, lifting weights, drinking protein shakes, eating apples.

My routine was basic. I thought of it as a matter of simple physics: If I burn more than I consume, my body will metabolize fat. It has to. I figured that at my weight, with my metabolism, I burned about 2,500 calories a day. So I kept to a 2,000-calorie diet and worked out like mad. Four runs a week (100 calories per mile), three swims (100 calories per 15 minutes), four weight sessions (300 calories an hour, plus beach mus-

▶▶MOVIES THAT MOTIVATE

Did *Rocky* and *The Karate Kid* inspire you to get physical? Of course they did—and it's okay to admit it. Here are a few other situations in which the right movie can prompt the right move

If you want to quit your job, watch *Animal House.*

At its heart, it's a manifesto against responsibility. Even if you don't quit tomorrow morning, at least bring a white horse into your boss's office tonight. It's a start.

If you want to get over the girl, watch *Swingers.*

Post-breakup Mike Peters (Jon Favreau) is pathetic, and you'll realize by the end of this movie that you're being pathetic, too. Pick yourself up and get back out there. You're so money, and you don't even know it.

If you want to grow a backbone, watch *Napoleon Dynamite.*

The lesson: Conformity is for losers. Embrace your passion and you'll never go wrong—even if that means wearing Moon Boots, blasting Jamiroquai, and dancing like a liger in public.

If you want to solve an integrity crisis, watch *The Insider.*

It's Pacino and Crowe's 157-minute pissing match to see who can do the right thing the hardest. More important, it's a reminder to always ask, Is this worth my good name?

If you want to serve a cold dish, watch *Walking Tall.*

The 1973 Joe Don Baker version. They mess with his family. They mess with his face. He brings them down with a bat. Send a message to your enemies: You will regret letting me live.

—MIKE ZIMMERMAN

cles). I made sure I never rang up more than a 7,000-calorie deficit (which equals 2 pounds of fat) in a given week, since your body freaks out when you do that.

NUMBER OF TIMES A YEAR MOST MEN SAY "I'M GOING TO GET BACK IN SHAPE!":

5 or more

It was tedious at first. The runs were painful, I was always sore, and it took so much damn time. I had to make a decision: The plan would come first—it was the only obligation I absolutely had to fulfill. Everything else in my life would have to fit in around it.

After about a month, after the initial shock had worn off, once my feet had calloused over and my hair had become ragged from the chlorine, the plan became something else. A dare. Not in the okay-tough-guy, No Fear, come-over-here-and-check-out-my-glutes kind of way. More like it was a daring thing to do.

Because, if you think about it, it's kind of absurd. Grown adults running through fields, unprompted, unchased, lifting heavy objects for no practical purpose, swimming back and forth repeatedly across a rectangle of water and heavy chemicals. It prompts a question in your mind, while you're pursuing these senseless tasks: What sort of creature does this kind of thing, anyway?

Over time, the answer becomes obvious, even if it's just something you feel in your bones: Because this is what I was born to do. This is what this body was made for.

As for that desk job, those hellishly vapid budget reports: Was I honestly made for that crap?

When the money that I'd saved ran out, I started working as a carpenter, walking around with a tool belt on all day, driving a 5-ton truck, familiarizing myself with the layout of Home Depot. It was good to be paid to sweat. The guys I worked with couldn't quite understand why I was doing basic construction instead of the cushy office job I'd left. "Hey, Stanford U," they'd say to me, "think you could nail this two-by-four into that frame over there? They teach you how to do that in school?"

The work itself had its benefits. At the end of the day, when my back hurt and my hands ached from pounding a hammer or wielding a screw gun for 8 hours, I felt as though I'd earned a drink. And anyway, there is a certain manful pride in knowing your way around a miter saw and a speed square. But it was mostly monotonous and nothing I had aspired to. I wasn't in it for that.

I was in it for the sense of possibility. For the idea that you can shake your life up like a soda bottle and smash it against the wall. That whatever prisons we construct in our lives—whether it's an awful job, a gut, an unhappy marriage, an addiction, the things in life that hem us in, that make us wake up in the morning in a cold sweat and think, How did I get like this? and How can I escape?—all these things are transient. For me, and maybe for anyone, the answer was, just leave. Tear the entire thing down.

In 6 months, I was down 55 pounds—to 170—and had all the accoutrements that so famously go with exercise: more energy, more confidence, better sleep, less stress. In place of the gut, I had the six-pack I'd had in college. I was also broke and single and had squandered what I had once understood to be a promising future. I didn't care.

I met a girl in Las Vegas. We exchanged phone numbers, and when I got back to Los Angeles, I called her. She invited me over to her place, a real dump in Culver City that was brimming with empty wine bottles and Liz Phair posters. When I walked in, she was sitting on the couch—skinny, big eyes, flat-chested, her shirt half unbuttoned, dirty blonde hair, and lots of eyeliner. My own private Marla Singer. I nearly cried.

"Have you seen this movie?" she asked, pointing to the television. And I couldn't even make this up: It was *Fight Club*—the scene where Ed Norton fakes a fight with his boss to get fired. In the process, he destroys the office, cutting his hands and back and face on the shattered glass of a coffee table. He walks out, whistling, pushing a pile of office equipment in a cart, with a smile on his face and blood dripping down his shirt. Fantastic.

I know, I know. Sophomoric. It is, a bit. But whatever the motivation, once I started taking exercise seriously, I felt more alive. I felt that my life had possibilities. I felt stronger. There's really nothing so basically transformative, nothing so regenerative, as getting in shape. Some of it is simple blood sugar, blood pressure, metabolism, and endorphins. When you're healthy, you feel better. Your high-school phys ed teacher could have told you that. But it's also the sense that if you can change your body, you can change anything. You feel your muscles working beneath your clothes, you become aware of your heartbeat, and you remember that you're an animal first and animals do not like to be fenced in.

The fact is, we're going to be dead someday, and I don't care how important we are or how much money we make, how refined our taste is in wine, music, clothes, literature, art, women. Those things are great, but there's just no escaping that your life begins and ends in your own body, your health, your ability to talk to That Girl with confidence, smile in the face of sobering news, senselessly lift heavy objects, swim great distances across various geometric figures, test your mortality, shatter some glass, eat an apple, tear across the plains, and run down a bloody gazelle.

It may be absurd, but honestly, you have to fill that void somehow, and you're simply not going to do it with muffin baskets.

THE EVER-EVOLVING WORKOUT

ADOPT ACTION HERO JASON STATHAM'S SECRETS OF
STRENGTH, SPEED, AND ALL-AROUND BADASSEDNESS
TO TURN YOUR WORLD UPSIDE DOWN

BY MIKE ZIMMERMAN

Jason Statham defines high metabolism. In fact, I'd bet he burned 500
calories in the time I spent talking to him. From his knuckle-popping
handshake (25 calories right there) to throwing shadow punches at my
face (another 38) to never quite sitting still as we spoke (a constant
7-calorie-per-minute simmer), he turns conversation into an anaerobic
workout.

Projecting physical strength is Statham's real magic—emphasis on
real. He was hustling black-market goods in London when he was type-
cast as a street thug in *Lock, Stock, and Two Smoking Barrels*. Now, the
38-year-old actor is known for the strong, silent skull-crackers he played
in *The Italian Job* and the *Transporter* films. In *Crank* he plays a crook
who will die if he doesn't keep his adrenaline inferno blazing. Which isn't
much of a stretch for Statham. He's in incredible physical condition—
everything he does is forceful—and his opinions are about as strong as
his handshake.

For one, he'll never hire a trainer. ("If you can't motivate yourself,
you're never going to get results.") He's built his physique through brutal intensity and ever-changing workouts designed to improve a skill—
whether it be platform diving for the British National Diving Team
back in the '90s or wushu staff fighting for *Transporter 2*.

But weight lifting just for the sake of heaving iron? Pointless, says
Statham. "Muscle-men grow on trees. They can tense their muscles and
look good in a mirror. So what? I'm more interested in practical strength
that's going to help me run, jump, twist, punch."

Here's how Statham builds a body that works.

FIX YOUR ATTITUDE FIRST

Statham's workout begins before he walks through a gym's front door. "I'm a firm believer in attitude," he says. "Some people just don't have that desire, and they need a good kick in the ass. Look, you've come to train here, let's f---ing train! Your body's like a piece of dynamite. You can tap it with a pencil all day, but you'll never make it explode. You hit it once with a hammer, bang! Get serious, do 40 hard minutes, not an hour and a half of nonsense. It's so much more rewarding."

> PERCENTAGE MORE CALORIES WALKING BACKWARD BURNS MORE THAN WALKING FORWARD:
> # 25

POUND YOUR CORE

Statham's buddy once dared him to do a marathon. He completed it in 3:51 (with virtually no distance training beforehand), and as a return dare, he challenged his pal to do the same abs workout Statham did back in his diving days. "We used to do 500 situp variations every day. Pike up with straight leg lifts and you'll strengthen your hip flexors, as well as your upper and lower abs." He notes with a grin that this workout made his friend "spew up."

HONE A SKILL AS YOU SWEAT

Statham is a monster fan of mixed martial arts—the grappling and striking you see in an Ultimate Fighting tournament. This training defines his "learn a skill" workout philosophy. A typical workout: "Shadow-boxing to warm up the back and shoulders," he says. Lunging and stretching for the legs. Next, five 3-minute rounds punching and kicking pads, then hitting the heavy bag for three rounds, and doing a session on the speed bag. He finishes with a circuit like the one described below.

USE YOUR OWN BODY WEIGHT

For explosiveness and reflexes, Statham has always used plyometrics. A fast, hard circuit requires no equipment. "I'll jump rope, then do squat thrusts, burpees [squat thrusts in which you leap instead of standing up], star jumps [from a crouch, jump up and spread your arms and legs into a star, and come back down into a crouch], pushups, tuck jumps [jump, lift legs, tuck], stepups." The key is explosive execution: "If I'm doing a pushup, I go down slowly and, bang, push up."

HAVE A PORTABLE WORKOUT

Even if Statham has only 20 minutes, he pulls no-gear, no-cost workouts from the manual in his head. One favorite came from his friend Bas Rutten, the mixed-martial-arts champion. "He uses punching combinations," Statham says. "He'll call out 'one'—a left. Then 'one, two'—a left, a right. Or 'three'—a left, a right, and a left hook. You can do that in a hotel room, anywhere." All you need is to bludgeon your excuses into a senseless heap. Just like Statham would.

GET MOVING

Men who don't begin exercising until later in life can still play catch-up with their heart health. In a German study of 300 people, those who started working out in their forties were half as likely to develop heart disease as the slugs who never sweated. That's nearly the same reduction realized by lifelong exercisers.

GET SOME MOTIVATION

A strong core doesn't just protect against injuries at the gym. A new study in the *American Journal of Public Health* shows that scrawny men are more likely to die in car crashes than their brawny brothers. Why? Hard muscle may shield a man's organs from damage during impact.

FEEL BETTER, FAST

For the first time, a study shows that moderate exercise immediately eases depression. Researchers from the University of Texas at Austin found that just one 30-minute bout of a moderately physical activity, such as walking, improved the moods of 40 patients with severe depression. After the walk, participants reported a 40 percent increase in feelings of well-being. Researchers say the emotional lift lasted about an hour.

GO HEAVY TO GET LIGHT

When researchers at the University of Southern Maine used an advanced method to estimate energy expenditure during exercise, they found that weight training burns as many as 71 percent more calories than originally thought. In fact, the researchers calculated that performing just one circuit of eight exercises can expend up to 231 calories. The more muscle you work, the more calories you'll burn, says study author Christopher Scott, PhD. Maximize the number of muscle fibers you activate in each set by performing a circuit in which you alternate upper-body movements with lower-body and abdominal exercises. This allows your upper-body muscles to rest while your lower-body muscles work, and vice versa—ensuring your best effort each set. Complete three full circuits of eight exercises, and it's likely you'll burn as many calories as you would by jogging for 30 minutes.

DOUBLE YOUR PLEASURE

Splitting your daily cardiovascular exercise into two sessions can double your stamina, according to new research from the University of New Hampshire. In the study, 37 men worked out either continuously for 30 minutes or in two 15-minute bouts. After 12 weeks, the twice-a-day group had improved their endurance by 21 percent—almost double the gain of the once-a-day group. Shorter workouts foster more intense exercise, which improves performance, say researchers.

MOVE IT TO LOSE IT

French researchers recently found that the secret to a flat belly isn't how many calories you burn; it's how often you burn them. When comparing total calories burned weekly, aerobic fitness level, and average exercise intensity in older men, the scientists discovered that those who simply spent the most time moving—regardless of the type of activity— had the leanest midsections. The magic numbers? Three to 4 days a week, accumulating a total of 4 hours.

SIGN ON THE DOTTED LINE

Would you pay $50 a month for better eyesight, a whiter smile, and a bigger bench press? A study in the *Journal of Sports Medicine and Physical Fitness* found that gym members work out longer and at higher intensities than people who don't have memberships. Health-club members are also 34 percent more likely to exercise regularly. Furthermore, they're almost three times likelier to have seen a general practitioner in the past year for regular checkups and are more inclined to visit a dentist, optometrist, or nutritionist. "People who are motivated to join a gym may also be more motivated toward preventive health," says the study's lead author, Elizabeth Ready, PhD. "Having paid for a membership and having a routine of attending at specific times could provide added motivation." Search "best gyms" at www.menshealth.com to find the perfect place to join.

MUSCLE-BUILDING SUPPLEMENT

Scientists have uncovered a new supplement that may help pack on muscle. In a recent report in *Strength and Conditioning Journal*, three recent studies show that the amino acid beta-alanine improves exercise performance. The mechanism? It helps ward off fatigue by improving a process known as carnosine synthesis.

"Beta-alanine is where creatine was in 1992," says Jeffrey Stout, PhD, CSCS, author of the report. "A couple of studies showed potential, but not enough to make solid recommendations." In the next couple of years, more research will be published on beta-alanine to help determine whether the amino acid deserves its early praise, says Stout. Until then, he suggests sticking with proven muscle-building supplements, such as creatine and whey protein.

CUSTOM-DESIGNED SHOES

Comfortable athletic shoes may be one step away. An English company, Prior 2 Lever, is using lasers to outfit professional soccer players with custom footwear. First, a laser scans the wearer's feet, then the athlete exercises while wearing a special insole that records the impact. Measurements of the foot, leg structure, and gait are taken. Working from 3-D blueprints, lasers fuse nylon particles into a shoe sole. The technology is expected to reach the United States in a few years.

SMART HEART RATE MONITOR

Fumbling with tiny watch buttons midrun ruins your momentum. That's why we love the Oregon Scientific SE102 action-oriented heart-rate monitor: Just tap the watch face to switch modes without breaking stride. It's a smart function we'd love to see on more pedigreed running computers. ($60. www.oregonscientific.com)

DRY-WICKING SHIRT

Quick-drying, sweat-wicking shirts are nothing new, but the Nike Sphere Dry won us over with its novel design. Sure, the well-placed vents kept our hot spots cool, and the reflective stripes meant we didn't worry about dodging cars on evening runs. But the nifty shoulder pouch sealed the deal by providing a jostle-free stash spot for keys and a hassle-free holster for both ear-bud cords and an iPod shuffle. ($35. www.nike.com)

ELECTRICITY-GENERATING BACKPACK

Bad news for Duracell: Lawrence Rome, PhD, a biology professor at the University of Pennsylvania, has invented a backpack that generates electricity. Springs on the pack use walking motion to power a generator, producing up to 7.4 watts—enough to run an MP3 player. Rome hopes to have the pack on the market in 2008.

GOLDEN RULES OF THE GYM

HEED THESE FIVE UNWRITTEN WORKOUT LAWS

1. **DON'T LEAVE DNA BEHIND:** Thirty-five percent of guys fail to wipe down machines after using them.

2. **DON'T GO BIG WITHOUT A SPOTTER:** Twenty-three percent of men have been pinned by a loaded barbell.

3. **MAINTAIN PROPER ORDER:** Sixteen percent of guys don't return dumbbells to their rightful spot

4. **STAY OFF GIRLY MACHINES:** Thirty percent of men use the inner- and outer-thigh machines

5. **FOLLOW THE "URINAL RULE":** Sixty-five percent of guys opt for the machine next to someone when others are open.

BURNING QUESTIONS

Testosterone peaks in the a.m.; is that when it's best to exercise?

While your T levels are highest in the morning, so is your risk for injuring your lower back, so we wouldn't say the a.m. is the best time to exercise. The problem has to do with your intervertebral disks— the cartilaginous shock absorbers between your vertebrae. As you sleep, the nuclei of the disks engorge with fluid, like ripe grapes ready to pop. If you stress your lower back when your disks are in this condition, you can tear them. Such herniated disks can take several weeks to heal. My advice: Wait at least 2 hours after waking before lifting weights, especially if your workout includes squats and deadlifts. By then, the fluid in your disks will be back to normal, and your risk of throwing out your back will be much lower.

Why do some guys' faces get so enormous as they age? William Shatner scares the hell out of me.

There are a lot of myths regarding why men gain weight in their faces, including excess alcohol consumption and the effects of aging. But really, it's all about genetics and weight gain. If you're predisposed to store fat in your face, then that's where it's going to go. Plus, the first place you notice weight gain is in your face, because it's your identity. William Shatner looks so puffy and pumpkinlike on *Boston Legal* because we remember how lean he looked in his *Star Trek* days.

"The good news is that the first place you gain weight is the first place you lose it," says Steven Aldana, PhD, a professor of lifestyle medicine in the College of Health and Human Performance at Brigham Young University in Provo, Utah. "You can lose weight in your face by reducing body fat, which means cleaning up your diet and increasing your physical activity."

So rather than choose plastic surgery, try losing pounds. For quick weight loss, start circuit training, a strength-training technique in which you move from exercise to exercise with no rest in between. Alternate upper-body movements (dumbbell chest presses, bent-over rows, hammer curls, triceps extensions) with lower-body and ab exercises (lunges, squats, crunches, back extensions). Complete three circuits of eight exercises three times per week with 1 minute rest between circuits.

Are there any benchmarks I can use to gauge my strength?

Everyone has a different physiology and fitness goal, and, therefore, his own "ideal" level of strength. But there are a few standards you can strive for: lifting one and a half times your body weight on the bench press, your body weight in a military press, and twice your body weight in a deadlift. More specific strength standards, however, are difficult to establish, especially if you use a sport like powerlifting as a benchmark. Powerlifters, after all, often use drugs and support gear to add tens or even hundreds of pounds to what they're able to shoulder. A top powerlifter who squats 900 pounds in full competition gear (weight belt, joint wraps) might manage only 700 "raw" pounds. The most important thing to remember is that if you can look in the mirror and feel strong, you probably are.

Can I gain muscle by weight training only twice a week? That's all I can fit in.

Absolutely. We recommend performing 4 to 6 compound movements (exercises that recruit several different muscle groups) using the "3-5 method." Do 3 to 5 sets of 3 to 5 repetitions, resting 3 to 5 minutes between sets. Sticking to a low rep count will allow you to lift more weight, maximizing your potential for growth in what little time you have.

Don't perform exactly the same moves in consecutive workouts. If you bench-press on day one, for example, do dumbbell presses the next. If you can fit in a third workout, do it, even if it consists of only one exercise. (Hint: Do squats.) Here's a sample week.

FIRST SESSION

1. Barbell squat: 5 sets of 3 reps per set; rest 3 to 5 minutes between sets

2. Chinup: 5 sets of 3 reps per set; rest 3 minutes between sets

3. Barbell bench press: 5 sets of 4 reps per set; rest 3 minutes between sets

4. Back extension: 5 sets of 4 to 5 reps per set; rest 3 minutes between sets

SECOND SESSION

1. Deadlift: 5 sets of 5 reps per set; rest 3 to 5 minutes between sets

2. Cable row: 5 sets of 5 reps per set; rest 3 minutes between sets

3. Dumbbell bench press: 5 sets of 5 reps per set; rest 3 minutes between sets

4. Military press: 5 sets of 4 to 5 reps per set; rest 3 minutes between sets

For exercise descriptions, visit www.bestlifeonline.com.

What's the best time to take protein supplements, before or after I lift?

You can't go wrong either way. But here's the best strategy: Consume protein both an hour before and immediately after your workout. Keep your preworkout protein shot simple—just a scoop of protein powder mixed with watered-down juice. Low Carb Grow! MRP ($23 for 3 pounds, www.t-nation.com) is a good choice. It's low in calories (110 per serving) and contains whey and casein, which provide your muscles with a time-released supply of protein.

In fact, a recent study at Baylor University found that men who consumed these milk proteins in combination gained 50 percent more muscle than men who consumed whey alone.

After you lift, make a shake using Surge by Biotest ($21 for 2 pounds, www.t-nation.com). Its 2-to-1 ratio of carbs to protein will provoke a surge of insulin that will help drive power-building amino acids into your muscles.

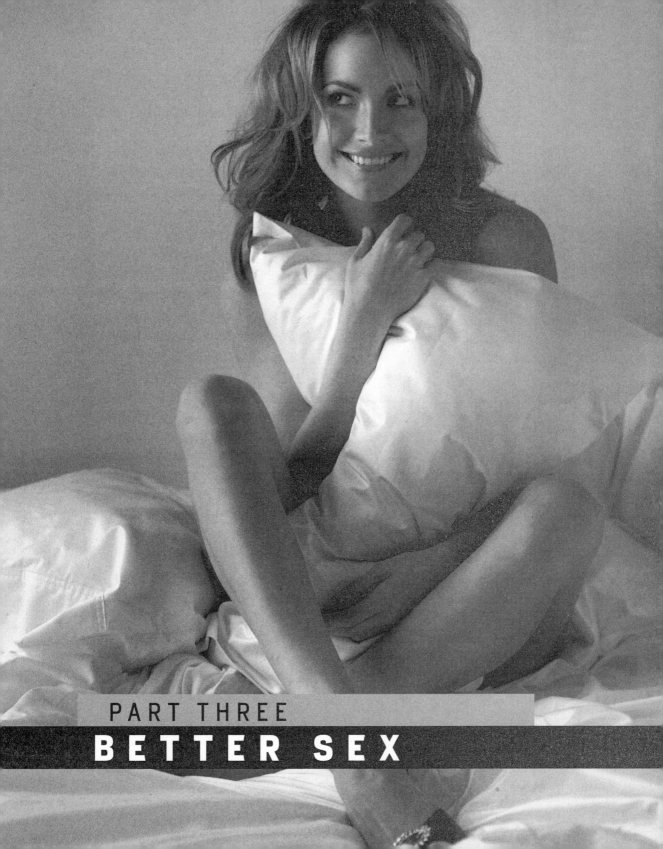

PART THREE
BETTER SEX

LOVE BITES

EAT THESE EIGHT FOODS TO FEEL
FRISKY FROM THE INSIDE OUT

BY MORGAN LORD

Sex-starved humans have been hunting get-in-the-mood grub for thousands of years. Romans slurped shellfish while splashing around public baths, and the Marquis de Sade downed untold quantities of Spanish fly as he boinked his way through 18th-century France. Of course, finding libido boosters with scientifically proven positive effects on sexual health is a different story (oysters, yes; Spanish fly, no). We tracked down eight foods that will increase hormone levels and get your blood pumping.

BANANAS

If you want sex to go the extra mile, fuel up for foreplay just as you would for a marathon. A big banana is the perfect food for bedroom endurance: Bananas contain B vitamins, which are key for converting carbohydrates into energy and are believed to help manufacture sex hormones such as testosterone. Munch on one a few hours before getting busy to make the most of your monkey business, says Hilda Hutcherson, MD, author of *Pleasure*.

CELERY

Eat celery sticks and you may suddenly seem completely irresistible. "Raw celery contains the male hormone androsterone, which can act as a pheromone to trigger female attraction," says Ava Cadell, PhD, author of *Passion Power*. After a few bites, your sweat glands start releasing the pheromone. If your girl seems too cranky to fool around, give her a stalk, too. Androsterone has mood-elevating effects in women, according to the *Journal of Fertility and Sterility*. Not a celery fan? Add a few truffle shavings to your meal. Truffles boast even more androsterone—enough for female pigs to detect the precious mushrooms growing as deep as 3 feet underground.

DARK CHOCOLATE

A recent Italian study found that women who report eating chocolate on a daily basis claim to have more satisfying sex lives. Coincidence? We think not. Willy Wonka's favorite raw material contains a cocktail of chemicals linked to relaxation, intoxication, and pleasure, Dr. Hutcherson says. Like other sweets, chocolate triggers the release of feel-good endorphins. It also provides small amounts of anxiety-quelling tryptophan, arous-

>>LOVE POTION

You don't need a PhD in biochemistry to know that a little alcohol can help you get in the mood. The cayenne pepper in this sexy cocktail contains capsaicin, which raises your heart rate and makes you sweat—simulating the physiological effects of sexual arousal.

RED-HOT MARTINI
1½ ounces Absolut Peppar Vodka, chilled
Splash grenadine
Cinnamon sugar

Combine vodka and grenadine in a shaker with ice. Run an ice cube around the rim of a martini glass, then place the glass rim-down on a plate sprinkled with cinnamon sugar. Set glass upright and strain in liquid.

ing caffeine, and a few substances—anandamide and theobromine—that, in large quantities, work like a psychedelic drug and an opiate, respectively. You'd have to down several pounds of chocolate to feel the funky effects, but simply nibbling a few squares after dinner will help transform your mood from stressed to saucy.

> **NUMBER OF PARTNERS FOR THE AVERAGE MAN IN HIS LIFETIME:**
> 1. BRAZIL: **11.37**
> 2. UNITED STATES: **8.77**
> 3. AUSTRALIA: **8.54**
> 4. UNITED KINGDOM: **8.28**
> 5. GREECE: **8.25**
> WORLD AVERAGE: **7.65**

FLAXSEEDS

Just 1 tablespoon of flaxseeds a day helps increase testosterone—the chemical with the most direct libido-boosting effect, according to Helen Fisher, PhD, author of *Why We Love*. Besides enhancing sex drive, these nutty-flavored seeds contain essential fatty acids, including omega-3 and omega-6, which are the major building blocks of all sex hormones. "If you don't have enough fatty acids, your hormone levels may decrease, and so will your desire," Dr. Hutcherson says. Flaxseed oil has twice the omega acids of fish, and 2 tablespoons of the seeds deliver 140 percent of your RDA. To rev your engine, either swallow a teaspoon of flaxseed oil or sprinkle a tablespoon of flaxseeds on your cereal and salads every day. Since both can spoil fast, get oil in opaque bottles and seeds in vacuum-sealed packs, which have longer shelf lives. If seeds aren't your thing, opt for walnuts, which contain about 90 percent of your omega RDA.

GINGER

Wondering what to cook for a special date? Make it an Asian stir-fry with loads of fresh ginger. The powerful root stimulates the circulatory system, increasing blood flow to the genitals. "Fresh ginger has a more pungent smell" than the stuff in a jar, Dr. Cadell says. So? Smelling ginger has a stronger effect on penile and vaginal blood flow than actually eating it. When a food or aroma raises blood pressure, vessels in the genitals admit a rush of blood that inflates erectile tissue. The vessels then close off, preventing blood from exiting the erogenous zones, keeping sensitivity levels high. Only powdered ginger on hand? It will also boost blood flow a bit, but the effect won't be as intense.

HONEY

No wonder newlyweds' sweaty getaways are called honeymoons. The sticky sweetener contains simple carbohydrates that provide instant energy and fuel for working muscles. "Honey is rich in B vitamins, which are needed for testosterone production, and it contains boron, which helps the body metabolize and use estrogen—an important part of blood flow and arousal," Dr. Hutcherson says. Use a few teaspoons as a natural sweetener in tea or spread it on toast with peanut butter.

NUTMEG AND CLOVE

Researchers have found that nutmeg and clove, both from evergreen trees, bolster the sexual activity of rats. Each stimulates the parasympathetic nervous system—helping the little critters, and you, relax—but the effects were greater with nutmeg. Just don't eat too much of the magical spice, as it also has hallucinogenic properties, Dr. Cadell says. A sprinkle on your cappuccino or hot cocoa should do the trick—as with chocolate, you'd have to eat a lot (about 2 tablespoons' worth on an empty stomach) before the walls would start melting.

OYSTERS

Ancient Romans pegged this shellfish as a sex-spurring food, and they were definitely onto something. Oysters contain high levels of zinc, a mineral required for the production of testosterone. A team of American and Italian researchers recently found that mussels, clams, and oysters deliver two types of amino acids that spark a rush of sex hormones. Be sure to chew your shellfish thoroughly before swallowing—you'll extract more of the mojo-cranking mineral.

THE LAWS OF ATTRACTION

BEEF UP YOUR SEDUCTIVENESS IN SIX EASY STEPS

BY DENNY WATKINS

Many things run through a woman's mind when you meet. Here's how to go from "hello" to "oh my."

YOUR APPROACH

Her brain quickly vets your height and facial symmetry the moment you meet. Now convince her of your character. Approach confidently; don't pretend to bump into her. "Men tend to talk to each other at angles to avoid confrontation," says Rutgers University anthropologist Helen Fisher, PhD, author of *Why We Love.* "But women face each other head-on and maintain eye contact."

YOUR INTRODUCTION

A good handshake isn't a shortcut to her bed, but a bad one can doom you. Hands are loaded with tactile nerves, and people with weak, clammy handshakes were perceived as shy and neurotic in a recent University of Alabama study. So hold your drink in your left hand and give her a firm but not bone-crushing grasp. Pay attention to her grip as well: The same study showed that women who give firmer handshakes tend to be more adventurous.

YOUR VOICE

The most attractive women prefer deep-voiced men, according to a recent study by Scottish researchers. It suggests high testosterone levels, a sign of strength and reproductive prowess. Push out air with your diaphragm, not your throat. This lengthens the column of air moving past your vocal cords. "It's like a built-in subwoofer," says voice coach Joanne Joella.

PERCENTAGE MEN WHO ENDED THEIR LAST RELATIONSHIPS:
39

YOUR ICEBREAKER

Say something that will draw out details about her. "Your friends seem nice—how did you get to know them?" is a compliment and a window into her past. Forming a bond will release dopamine, a mood booster in her brain. Show off your interest with verbal nods of agreement ("uh-huh," "go on"), adds Alex Pentland, PhD, an MIT professor who designed software that assesses whether speed daters are feeling sparks.

YOUR CONVERSATION

We all know to ask lots of questions and to avoid flat-out boasting. But don't sell yourself short. "Women listen very carefully for signs of status and wealth," says Dr. Fisher. Keep any references to financial or personal success oblique, though; let her curiosity draw out the details. Another crucial conversation tip: Talk at the same pace she does, and she'll consider you intelligent, kind, confident, and ambitious, according to a University of Maryland study.

YOUR BODY LANGUAGE

Attraction causes couples to mirror each other's body language. But don't be overeager to connect. Stay relaxed and let her set the tone, says Lisa Clampett, founder of the Matchmaking Institute. Fidgeting conveys nervousness and triggers the empathetic release of stress chemicals in her brain. "Once she brushes your shoulder or thigh, reciprocate within a minute or two," Fisher says. Or touch her inner forearm, a nerve-rich zone that will create sparks.

YOUR DEAL CLOSER

If you've made the right sort of first impression, she might be wondering how you are in bed. "Consciously or not," says Dr. Fisher, "she's looking for signs that you're patient and sensitive to the ways her body finds pleasure." So handle the darts delicately. Call out the scent notes of a bottle of wine. Show refined tastes in these areas and she'll suspect you have others worth exploring—back at her place.

THE 12 STAGES OF SEDUCTION

USE THIS GUIDE TO WOO ANY WOMAN, ANYTIME

BY LAUREN MURROW

We asked 1,000 women to chart the course from first impression to the morning after. Here's what they said.

WHAT'S THE BEST WAY TO ASK HER OUT?

Fifty-three percent of women say: Forget the gimmicks. A casual but straightforward phone call or conversation is the way to go: "I think you're great. Let's have dinner. You free on Friday?"

"Be direct and call it a date," says Caroline Tiger, author of *How to Behave: Dating and Sex*. "You'll set the tone from the beginning." Avoid projecting smarmy confidence, adds Amy DeZellar, a self-confessed "serial dater" and a blogger at www.datingamy.com. "Too-suave come-ons are instant weed-out cues for women." Remember: You're confident, but not that she'll say yes. Cold feet? Your invite doesn't have to be a formal one. Twenty-six percent of women said it's fine to pop the question into another conversation.

DATING DON'T: Only 7 percent of women want to be asked out by way of a note, mix CD, or, God forbid, boom-box serenade.

HOW TO RECOVER: More than 49 percent of women with "other plans" aren't just feeding you a line—they want you to ask again, right away. Mind the gap between a bona fide conflict and a polite blow-off: "Blow-offs are all about why she can't do something," says one respondent. "If she likes you, she'll mention that she's free another night, or propose her own idea."

HOW DO YOU SEGUE FROM DINNER TO A MORE INTIMATE ENCORE?

Fifty-four percent of women say: Find a natural sequel to dinner. Successful seduction requires ratcheting up the intimacy in stages, not jumping

**AVERAGE LENGTH OF
FOREPLAY, IN MINUTES:**
1. **UNITED KINGDOM: 17.44**
2. **AUSTRALIA: 17.20**
3. **GERMANY: 16.92**
4. **MEXICO: 16.91**
5. **CZECH REPUBLIC: 16.43**
6. **UNITED STATES: 16.42**
WORLD AVERAGE: 15.78

from tapas to topless. After you've broken the ice—over drinks, appetizers—it's time for the main event. "That's when the question of physical intimacy comes into play," says Diane Mapes, author of *How to Date in a Post-Dating World*. So find someplace intimate. "It's like a chemistry lab," agrees DeZellar. "It's hard to test your compatibility in a place like Starbucks that's so bright, loud, and corporate." The litmus test: Graze her hand or rest your palm on the small of her back; she should return the favor within 5 minutes.

DATING DON'T: Inviting her to your place too quickly.

HOW TO RECOVER: Recovering a conversational fumble is simple. Laugh at yourself; move on. "No one is perfect. She'll appreciate it if you show you know how to defuse the awkwardness," says David Matalon, coauthor of *The Concise Guide to Sounding Smart at Parties*. "You're only doomed when you dwell."

WHAT'S THE BEST WAY TO ASK HER BACK TO YOUR PLACE?

Fifty-one percent of women say: Let's take it one step at a time. Honesty can be refreshing, but a straightforward seduction can backfire. "If he says, 'I want you to come back to my place,' it's understood that I'm coming back to be intimate with him," says Amber Madison, author of *Hooking Up: A Girl's All-Out Guide to Sex and Sexuality*. "That might work with some women, but it can be a turnoff for others. But if he invites me up for a drink, I can feel out the vibe. Sometimes he needs to prove himself before I decide I'm going to get physical." Watch for subtle signs of attraction before making the invite. "Look for gestures, like if I hold your arm when walking back to the car after dinner," says one respondent. If you're uncertain, let her choose between a nightcap at your place or at a neutral location.

DATING DON'T: Brutal honesty. Telling her you want to get close to her and that you don't want the night to end.

YOU HAVE 5 MINUTES TO QUICKLY CLEAN YOUR PLACE. WHAT DO YOU HIT?

Sixty-seven percent of women say: The cleanliness of your bathroom is paramount. "Once I'm at his house, I'm 75 percent ready," says one woman surveyed, "unless his bathroom is filthy." "You should care enough to clean before she arrives," says Mapes. Outside of your bathroom, make sure to point out photos of your travels or of family and friends. "They make you look warm and connected, not like the guy from *American Psycho*," says DeZellar. They're also conversation starters. One caveat: Keep Mom's mug out of the bedroom.

DATING DON'T: Making sure your bedroom looks inviting to her.

HOW TO RECOVER: Bedroom look more like a brothel? Keep it clean, not cocky. Ditch the rose petals and the phalanx of scented votives for one new candle. Anything more looks presumptuous.

WHEN DO YOU MAKE YOUR FIRST MOVE?

Seventy percent of women say: Let me have a chance to talk and relax first. Only 22 percent of the women we polled said they'd like your first move to be a spontaneous peck at the bar, at the restaurant, or even on your front steps. And "if you kiss me as soon as we walk in the door, you'll make me feel sleazy," says one woman. Let the mood marinate for at least 15 minutes. "Treat her like a guest—offer her a drink and turn on some music or entertainment," says Tiger. "You want the date vibes to transition naturally into hooking up." When you're setting the mood, forgo the Sex Pistols for something mellow but passionate, such as the Shins, Coldplay, or U2. Researchers at Florida State University found that playing music can significantly decrease symptoms of stress; 54 percent of women confirmed they're charmed by the vanilla crooning of Mr. Gwyneth Paltrow.

DATING DON'T: As soon as we're inside—in the elevator or once we get in the door.

HOW DO YOU MAKE THE FIRST MOVE?

Thirty-eight percent of women say: Make your move after our bodies have synced. Planting the first kiss is a high-wire act. One warning sign she's not ready to jump: "She'll be chattering and desperately try-ing to fill the silences," says DeZellar. "Your bodies should have a chance to synchronize. It can't be a sneak attack." If she's seated, ask her to help you mix a drink or drop a dollop of syrup onto a sundae—anything to bring her upright and near. Stow the tongue helicopter: Sixty-one percent of women prefer a kiss that's short and sweet. "Kiss gently around her mouth, face, neck, and ears," suggests Jennifer Worick, author of *Worst Case Scenario Survival Handbook: Dating and Sex*. If she increases the intensity, follow her lead.

DATING DON'T: I crack a joke to disarm her.

HOW TO RECOVER: What to do if you pick the wrong moment? Lend some levity to the situation: "Sorry, maybe that wasn't the best time to maul you." Nearly half of all of women said they're up for another attempt, even if you chose a bad moment the first time.

HOW DO YOU KNOW IF SHE'S READY TO TRANSITION TO SOMETHING MORE SERIOUS?

Fifty percent of women say: Pay attention to my passion levels. They're your traffic signals. "Most women assume men have no problem going farther," says Worick, "so they'll make the move, if they're comfortable." Let the intensity escalate naturally, looking for subtle (or not-so-subtle) invitations. Firmer kisses and increasingly forceful caresses signal when she's ready to speed up. Drive by her breasts or hips with your hands and gauge her reaction—if she tenses, shift into neutral; if she coos, hug the curves. Once you've crossed the equator—above or below the clothes—you have the green light to relocate to your bedroom. "Take her by the hand, pull her up, and lead her there," says Worick.

DATING DON'T: I wait for her to tell me what to do; women shouldn't be afraid to ask for what they want.

WHAT'S YOUR FOREPLAY GAME PLAN?

Sixty-eight percent of women say: Warm me up slowly. Intimate mas-sages are passé. "It's so transparent," says Madison. "It's obviously just a way to initiate contact and get into her pants." The same goes for rose petals between the sheets or a sea of tea lights in the bedroom. "Women develop really sensitive radar for cheesiness," says Tiger. Keep it simple: Spend at least 10 minutes kissing and caressing before trying to rid her of those pesky clothes. Rub her body through the fabric and lightly graze your fingers along her breasts and thighs to build anticipation of what's to come. The better you build her up now, the more passionate the payoff will be.

PERCENTAGE OF MEN WHO ENDED THEIR LAST RELATIONSHIPS: 39

DATING DON'T: I try to move things along in under 10 minutes.

WHAT'S THE BEST WAY TO START UNDRESSING A WOMAN?

Seventy-four percent of women say: Quid pro quo—we'll help each other disrobe. One-sided strip shows sacrifice the most automatic sort of foreplay: the slow reveal. "If a woman ends up naked too quickly, she suddenly feels vulnerable and awkward," says Madison. Instead of fixating on her breasts or fumbling with her pants, divert your attention to underappreciated bare body parts. As you undress her, use your hands, then follow with your lips and tongue, lingering around hot spots like her neck, abdomen, and inner thighs. "Make it into a teasing game," says Worick. "Always touch her most sensitive parts last. And take the time to admire each layer of undress."

DATING DON'T: I remove her clothes for her.

HOW TO RECOVER: Halting the southern march of your hands or lips doesn't mean she's asking you to call off the entire campaign. "When things start quickly, there's nowhere to go but, uh, down," says Worick. So regroup. Turn down the intensity, then build back to sensual kissing and caressing."

WHAT'S YOUR GOAL FOR FIRST-TIME SEX?

Forty-five percent of women say: Increase my feeling of closeness. Stash the Kama Sutra, Ron Jeremy. Women aren't looking for a freak show the first time. "It's not even crucial that she climax," says Madison. "He has to be gentle, passionate, and tuned in to what makes her feel good." Pause to breathe and reestablish eye contact between kisses, and make her feel sexy by conveying your pleasure. More than 83 percent of women prefer the missionary position the first time. "If she's on top, she has to worry about whether she's going too fast or too slow," says Madison. Vary your rhythm according to the urgency of her response. The better she feels, the less guarded the sex will become.

DATING DON'T: The more orgasmic, the better: I want her to have an unforgettable, over-the-top experience.

HOW DO YOU COMMUNICATE DURING SEX?

Forty-four percent of women say: Pay attention to my body language. "Describing sexual wants and needs doesn't come naturally to most people. Women don't want to reveal their sexual fantasies the first time," says Madison. More than 39 percent of women, in fact, said too much talking was their biggest sexual turnoff. Instead, watch for signs of physical arousal, like groans or more forceful or faster body movements, to know when you've hit the spot.

DATING DON'T: I ask her questions to make sure I'm pleasing her at all times.

WHAT DO YOU SAY WHEN PARTING IN THE MORNING?

Eight-two percent of women say: Tell me you want to see me again—and soon. A proper parting line includes specifics. Don't just say you'll call; tell her you'll call this afternoon, then deliver. Better yet, book her for next Saturday: Eighty-two percent of women prefer to nail down another date before you go. "It validates that there was an emotional connection as well as a physical spark," says Mapes, "whereas 'I'll call you later' is code for 'Goodbye and good luck.'" In fact, more than 57 percent of women said they want to hear from you again the same day. "Women equate the time it takes you to pick up the phone with your level of interest," says Mapes. "The sooner you call, the more sparks you felt."

DATING DON'T: "I had fun, thanks."

HOW TO RECOVER: Left with a lackluster farewell? You have a 1-hour window to recover your fumble. Call her cell and book a repeat.

PLEASURE: AROUND THE WORLD

LEARN THE SEX SECRETS OF 40,000 MEN IN 42 COUNTRIES

BY LAURA ONGARO AND MATT BEAN

When it comes to wooing women, men aren't perfect. But perhaps guys are more selfless than their rep suggests. *Men's Health* asked readers from all 35 international editions—our largest global survey ever—what sexual skills they'd most like to improve. The most common answers: seducing a woman more effectively and bringing her to orgasm every time. Of course, there's another way to read this. It could be that men from Argentina to Ukraine simply realize that our pleasure rises and falls with hers—that by stoking her fires, they'll have hotter sex more often. To that end, we interviewed hundreds of women and sex experts from around the globe. The result is what follows: an expert lesson in the universal language of lust.

MAKE IT EASY FOR HER

You catch her eye from across the room. Now what? "Playing games wastes everyone's time," says Nikki Hayia, sex editor at *Men's Health* Greece. "Women prefer a man who knows what he wants, especially if what he wants is us." Use body positioning to advertise your confidence, suggests Helen Fisher, PhD, a research professor in the anthropology department at Rutgers University in New Jersey. If you're sitting, keep an open position—legs apart, head up, chest out, back straight. If you're standing, position your shoulders toward her while turning your head toward your conversational partner. Mirror her actions to signal your attention—when she drinks, you drink. When she changes her body position, so do you. If you see that you and she are moving in tandem, to a beat, then it's time to make your move. "I know whether I'm attracted to you, so I don't need a pickup line," says Sara, a 28-year-old bartender in South Africa. "Just introduce yourself."

**NUMBER OF TIMES PER
WEEK THE AVERAGE
MAN HAS SEX:**
 1. **KOREA: 4.50**
 2. **GREECE: 4.20**
 3. **ROMANIA: 4.08**
 4. **PHILIPPINES: 3.95**
 5. **RUSSIA: 3.87**
 . . .
17. **UNITED STATES: 2.95**
WORLD AVERAGE: 2.80

CRAFT AN INVITATION THAT WORKS

"A woman who's dressed to thrill is less likely to go home with you," says Emily Dubberley, a British sex expert and the author of *Brief Encounters: The Woman's Guide to Casual Sex.* "You don't want to be the third of 25 guys to approach her that evening." Instead, go for the woman in the background. "She's with a friend or two, both of whom are brighter, brasher, and louder than she is," says Dubberley. And remember: "A woman needs to feel as though it's a passionate one-off, not planned," says Pam Spurr, a United Kingdom–based sex expert and the author of *Sinful Sex: The Uninhibited Guide to Erotic Pleasure.* This depends on how you ask her to come home with you. "Coffee at my place?" is too stark a transition, because it suggests the party's ending. Instead, try "I've got a bottle of wine in the fridge at home—could we carry on this conversation back there?" This suggests a continuation of the fun. "It's honest and exciting, and the notion of a man with wine in the fridge is encouraging," says Spurr. "Make sure you have fresh towels in the bathroom and clean sheets on your bed, too."

SEDUCE HER EARLY AND OFTEN

Foreplay is like an investment. Start early—way before her clothes come off—and you'll reap greater rewards. "The longer we wait, the better our orgasm," says Spurr. Begin your wooing when she's unattainable—you're both at work; she's stuck in traffic; her father just asked you to pass the salt. "It could be a sexy e-mail or a voice mail or just a smile," says Birgit Ehrenberg, a sex columnist in Germany. "The important thing is that you're building the tension." Once you're together, pay attention to the details. "Instead of making a beeline for her breasts, try tugging on her hair while you kiss her, exhaling near her ear, or just gently kissing her eyelids," says Caroline Hurry, a sex writer in South Africa. "For women, a combination of boldness and tenderness is crucial."

AWAKEN ALL HER SENSES

Nearly 30 percent of the men we surveyed wish they were better—and quicker—at seducing women. Here's the secret: Because arousal has a cumulative effect, try to engage at least three of her senses at a time. As Marta, a 27-year-old Italian lawyer told us, "It takes time and lots of ingredients—smells, tastes, sounds—to heat us up." The next time you're near a mirror, pull her close and let her have the full view as you kiss her neck and caress her body, suggests Sonia Parreira Duque, a clinical psychologist in Lisbon. "Or play her favorite record, spritz her favorite fragrance around the bedroom, and leave some small pieces of fruit and chocolate beside the bed." One no-fail move: Give her the spa treatment. "Choose a fragrant shampoo and swirl your fingertips around her scalp with the warm, sudsy water," says Spurr. "The massage and fragrance will help her relax, unleashing oxytocin, a feel-good hormone that promotes emotional bonding." Next step: physical bonding.

LAST LONGER IN BED

"There's a Hungarian proverb that says, 'Do not paint the devil on the wall, for it will appear,'" says Agnes Beregszászi, a sex columnist in Hungary. Translation: The area of the brain responsible for triggering orgasm is engaged whether you're trying to have one or halt one. The more attention you pay to your orgasm, the more likely it is to arrive. So concentrate on gauging your partner's response to each move instead—did she "oooh" or "ehh"?—until you find her sweet spot. "Good sex is like driving to a faraway city," says Beregszászi. "You know your destination, but you need to concentrate on the road ahead of you—turn left here, turn right there. If you focus on what's happening now—her silky thighs on your hips, say—you can diffuse your pleasure through-out your whole body." Oh, and she'll love it: "When my boyfriend slows down, I feel every bit of him," says Petra, a 30-year-old receptionist in Belgium. "It helps me focus on the sensation, and really puts me over the top when he begins to speed up again."

TEST-DRIVE A HOT FOREIGN IMPORT

The least-pleasing position for women—missionary—is still the go-to move for 48 percent of American men and 42 percent of men worldwide.

You can do better. These sex positions span the Earth, and might just make it move.

SPAIN—THE DOWNWARD DOG: Ask her to rest her chest on the bed while lifting her rear in the air. From your knees, enter her from behind. Thrust downward slightly and the bottom of your penis will massage her vaginal wall where her G-spot is located. "This position lengthens her vaginal wall," says Pedro Otero, a sexologist in Spain, "which tightens her and makes you feel bigger."

INDIA—THE FUSION: Sit on the bed or floor with your legs extended out in front of you. Lean back about 15 degrees, supporting yourself with your arms. Ask her to sit facing you, and help her lower herself on your penis while she leans back and supports her body with her arms behind her. Her knees should be bent and near your shoulders.

"This is one of the few positions in which the union of sexual organs is visible for both partners," says Mahinder Watsa, MD, a sex therapist in India. "That translates into an increase in sexual excitement."

BRAZIL—THE AMAZON: Lie on your back with your knees to your chest. Ask her to squat on your erection, facing you, one foot on each side of your abdomen and her thighs resting on yours. Wrap your legs around her waist and hold hands to help her balance. "This is perfect for women who aren't strong enough to be on top for a long time," says Laura Muller, a sex advisor in Brazil and the author of *500 Questions on Sex*. "It lets her control penetration and leaves one of your hands free to caress her clitoris."

HUNGARY—THE LAZY LADY: In a spooning position (you're on the outside, holding yourself up by your elbow), ask her to raise her top knee; then enter her from behind. The angle of penetration will stimulate her G-spot while your hand plays gently with her clitoris. "Your chest will be hugging her back," says Beregszászi, "so you can match your breathing and rhythm, and thus be lulled into a very gentle, intimate togetherness." And what woman could say no to that?

GET ADDICTED TO LOVE

Blood samples have revealed biochemical evidence that intense romantic love fades after a year in a new relationship, according to a recent study in the journal *Psychoneuroendocrinology*. Researchers tested the blood of 58 men and women who reported being newly and madly in love and compared the blood with samples from people in long-lasting relationships. They looked at levels of nerve growth factor (NGF), believed to be a mediator of anxiety, emotions, and behaviors. Higher NGF levels corresponded to reportedly intense feelings of passionate love. And levels were nearly double in the new lovers, compared with those in long-term partnerships.

"Love is not only poetry; it also has a strong biological basis," says Enzo Emanuele, MD, of the University of Pavia, in Italy. "An adage says that 'love is an addiction.' Perhaps we may become tolerant of our partner, though nevertheless remaining 'addicted.'"

THINK, HARD

Bill Clinton learned this too late: Research shows that when men have an erection, they're more open to unusual, deviant, or illegal sex acts and behaviors, reports the *Journal of Behavioral Decision Making*. In the study, 35 college men rated their interest in certain acts when they were not aroused, and then again—at least a day later—while they had an erection. The men rated their interest on a scale from zero for "no" to 100 for "yes," with 50 being "possibly." The unflattering averages:

Research Question	Appeal when not aroused	Appeal when aroused
Could you enjoy having sex with someone you hated?	53	77
If an attractive woman proposed a threesome with a man, would you do it?	19	34
Could it be fun to have sex with someone who is extremely fat?	13	24
Would you encourage a date to drink to increase your chances for sex?	46	63
Would you tell a woman you loved her to increase your chances?	30	51
Can you imagine having sex with a 50-year-old woman?	28	55
Would you find it exciting to be spanked by an attractive woman?	50	68

DITCH THE HEADACHE MEDICINE

Could over-the-counter painkillers affect your erection? A study published in the *Journal of Urology* says nonsteroidal anti-inflammatory drugs (NSAIDs) such as aspirin, ibuprofen, and naproxen may weaken your ability to get and keep an erection. The survey of 1,126 men ages 50 to 70 found that erectile dysfunction was about twice as common in men who regularly took the painkillers as in those who didn't. The researchers speculate that NSAIDs may interfere with the production of nitric oxide, a process that's crucial to erections.

Don't panic yet—more research is needed to determine if the effect is the same in younger men, says Rahman Shiri, MD, the study's lead researcher, of the University of Tampere, in Finland.

PERCENTAGE OF MEN WHO'VE TAKEN A PERFORMANCE-ENHANCING PILL:
1. UNITED STATES: **21%**
2. UNITED KINGDOM: **15%**
3. SOUTH AFRICA: **14%**
4. THE NETHERLANDS: **12%**
5. PHILIPPINES: **12%**
WORLD AVERAGE: **11%**

BE SAFE

Syphilis cases have increased among Americans for the fourth straight year, in part because of a rise in Internet-solicited sex, according to the Centers for Disease Control and Prevention. Men are six times more likely than women to be diagnosed with the disease.

SPERM'S STARTING GUN

New research at Harvard medical school may help in the development of a male contraceptive and aid in the treatment of infertility. Scientists isolated a protein believed to be the key to sperm's swimming action, or motility. Sperm without the protein (known as CatSper) were nearly immobile, according to a study in *Nature*. "This may lead to a way to diagnose male infertility," says researcher David Clapham, MD, PhD. Plus, researchers are studying a male contraceptive that would block the protein.

MOOD SETTER

Made from cosmetic-grade soy wax and natural plant extracts, the Ember Natural Emollient Massage Candle sets just the right mood and lets you get your glow on for 60 hours. Drip a little body-friendly wax on her skin and you'll really fire her up. ($48. www.jimmyjane.com)

MALE CONTRACEPTION

The times they are a changin'. In bed. In September 2006, researchers began a 90-man study of the Intra Vas Device (IVD), a contraceptive for you. During the procedure, doctors insert two sets of silicone plugs into the narrow tube called the vas deferens—the one sperm use to get from the testes to the penis. The first plug stops sperm midjourney. The second catches any squirmers that squeeze past the first. The procedure is reversible, but the plugs should last a lifetime. Which is about how long the wait will feel: The IVD probably won't be available in the United States until 2010.

AVERAGE NUMBER OF TIMES PER WEEK A MAN MASTURBATES:
1. PHILIPPINES: **5.65**
2. UNITED KINGDOM: **5.53**
3. BRAZIL: **5.32**
4. FRANCE: **5.29**
5. MALAYSIA: **5.27**
. . .
12. UNITED STATES: **4.13**
WORLD AVERAGE: **4.30**

IPOD HEADPHONE SPLITTER

PERCENTAGE OF MEN WHO'VE NEVER CHEATED WITH ANOTHER WOMAN:
1. POLAND: **63%**
2. GERMANY: **62%**
3. AUSTRALIA: **60%**
4. THE NETHERLANDS: **59%**
5. UNITED KINGDOM: **57%**
6. UNITED STATES: **52%**
WORLD AVERAGE: **50%**

Sitting on a plane, sprawling on a beach blanket, cuddling in that giant hammock—wouldn't it be more fun and romantic to do these things listening to the same tunes or book on tape instead of zoning out in separate worlds? Plug the Belkin Headphone Splitter ($4. www.belkin.com) into your iPod and suddenly it's possible. Bonus: Every song you associate with hanging out together has the potential to improve your sex life. According to a 2004 study in the *Personality and Social Psychology Bulletin*, reminding each other of shared experiences ramps up desire. So when you hear "Clocks" by Coldplay, say "Honey, remember that time we . . ."

SPEAK HER BODY LANGUAGE

FIVE WAYS TO MEET WOMEN, USING SOME
COMMON SENSE AND YOUR OWN SPECIAL FLAIR

1. **WATCH FOR THE HEAD FAKE:** Don't misread a glance as an invitation. A woman could be scanning the room for friends or, worse, her 260-pound boyfriend. If she really wants to send a message, she'll let you catch her peeking. If she's bold—on the prowl, even—she'll make eyes. If she's demure, she'll simply glance at you, then leave her head pointed in your direction while she returns to her conversation.

2. **STAND UP STRAIGHT:** After your initial approach, her brain will work out a bit of math to see how you match up. Parallel her body language to avoid coming on too strong. Don't mirror her exact movements; just match her physical tone. If she's animated, you're animated. If she's subdued, so are you. Avoid aggressive postures— hand on cocked hip, legs apart, or torso lowered in a three-point stance, shoulder pads pointed at her solar plexus—and you won't trip her stalker sensor.

3. **WEAR DOWN THAT WALL:** Quit clutching that drink in front of you like it's your lifeline. Barriers help in business, but not when making new friends. If you can't set the drink down, hold it at your left side, keeping your right hand warm and inviting for introductions.

4. **SET THE TABLE:** Bar tables are like wingmen. Square tables create a barrier that can comfort a woman if you're approaching her for the first time. Circular tables create a more intimate feel by removing the edges or boundaries between you.

5. **STOP LISTENING:** She seems rapt, but how to know if she's really interested? Look for the head cock. Like a puppy, she'll lean her head toward her shoulder, putting her neck in a vulnerable position. That means she trusts you. And remember: A real smile shows in the eyes as well as the cheeks.

PERCENTAGE OF MEN WHO'D PAY ANYTHING TO PLEASE A WOMAN:
1. INDONESIA: **64%**
2. PORTUGAL: **51%**
3. POLAND: **42%**
4. THE NETHERLANDS: **40%**
5. ITALY: **39%**
. . .
22. UNITED STATES: **19%**
WORLD AVERAGE: **31%**

PERCENTAGE OF MEN WHO'VE HAD A THREESOME:
1. BRAZIL: **20%**
2. UNITED KINGDOM: **17.6%**
3. AUSTRALIA: **17.5%**
4. UNITED STATES: **17%**
5. RUSSIA: **15%**
WORLD AVERAGE: **14%**

BURNING QUESTIONS

Are there any exercises I can do that might help me last longer?

You've probably heard about Kegel exercises, but most guys do them wrong. For the full effect, you need to isolate your pelvic-floor muscles (the same ones you squeeze to stop the flow of urine midstream) and keep your abs and glutes out of the picture. Squeeze the pelvic muscles for 10 seconds, then release; if you're doing it right, it should be unnoticeable to the casual observer, which means no gyrating butt cheeks or clenched abs. Put in 5 minutes a day doing this covert routine and your lady will thank you.

What's the best sexual position to make my new girlfriend happy?

Assuming she's confident in her body and skills, woman-on-top works best. "It'll be more fun for her, and most women will be more orgasmic in that position" because they can control their stimulation, says *Men's Health* sex columnist Debby Herbenick, PhD. But for your first time together, go with missionary, modified. Place your chest at her shoulders, allowing your pubic bone to rub against her clitoral area.

How can I be more than a spectator when my girlfriend is on top?

It's all in the hips: Grab her by her sides and pull her toward your abdomen, syncing your rhythm and increasing pressure on her clitoris. You can also deliver a playful slap to her derriere, gently touch her breasts, or, if she leans in close, crunch upward to kiss her nipples. Meanwhile, focus on your own arousal—savor the sensation, but relax your pelvis to increase your staying power.

Our sex life is great, but I want to surprise my girlfriend. What erogenous zones might I have missed?

Any place on her body where the nerve endings are close to the surface is a good bet, like the back of her knees, the inside of her arms, or even her fingertips. Gently brush the tips of your fingers across her torso, tenderly kissing the inside of her thighs, or lightly caress her palms. Some women find it erotic to have their fingers and toes kissed. You've probably already found that she loves to have her lower back massaged. Kneading it can relax and arouse at the same time. The perineum—the area between the vagina and the anus—often goes unexplored. It's extremely sensitive to even the lightest touch.

> **NUMBER OF POSITIONS IN THE AVERAGE MAN'S SEXUAL ARSENAL:**
> 1. HUNGARY: **8.27**
> 2. ARGENTINA: **5.76**
> 3. SPAIN: **4.63**
> 4. BRAZIL: **3.95**
> 5. GREECE: **3.83**
> . . .
> 16. UNITED STATES: **2.78**
> WORLD AVERAGE: **3.35**

I'm always drenched in sweat when I have sex with my wife, but she freezes if I pull back the covers. Any advice?

Hot sex doesn't have to mean sweaty sex. She'll warm up faster if she's on top doing the work. Wrap her in a sheet till she's warm. The downward dog position (see page 92) is another way to keep her warm—you're the blanket.

I thought my testicles were just reproductive organs. So why does it feel so good when a girl plays with them?

Since they're so important, your testicles have a built-in alarm system of nerve endings that are sensitive to both pleasure and—as men well know—intense pain. If ball play drives you wild but you're trying to last longer, switch to a position that takes the testicles away from the action, like woman on top and leaning forward. Otherwise, enjoy the ride.

My wife says my semen irritates her vagina. Could it be something I ate?

There's a small chance your semen could be too acidic. About 30 percent of ejaculate is acidic prostate fluid, balanced by alkaline secretions from the seminal vesicles. Before seeing your doctor, though, I'd rule out any chemical products as the cause of the irritation. If the pain remains, she should ask her doctor to check for an infection or hypersensitivity to semen.

Is there anything wrong with taking Viagra if I don't need it?

Viagra works by increasing bloodflow to the penis. If everything is in working order, Viagra won't help; it's not an aphrodisiac or a magical stamina booster. Besides the headaches and painfully persistent erections (you can have too much of a good thing), doctors also worry that men may develop a psychological dependence on medication they don't need, eventually making it difficult to maintain an erection without the drug. Bottom line: No plumbing problems, no point. Drugs like Viagra help many men, but it's best to wait until you need them.

PERCENTAGE OF MEN WHO'VE HAD A ONE-NIGHT STAND:
1. PORTUGAL: **81%**
2. BRAZIL: **77%**
3. AUSTRALIA: **65%**
4. RUSSIA: **64.7%**
5. UNITED STATES: **61%**
WORLD AVERAGE: **59%**

PERCENTAGE OF MEN WHO'VE PAID FOR SEX:
1. KOREA: **42%**
2. BRAZIL: **34%**
3. PHILIPPINES: **32%**
4. GREECE: **31%**
5. RUSSIA: **26%**
...
18. UNITED STATES: **17%**
WORLD AVERAGE: **21%**

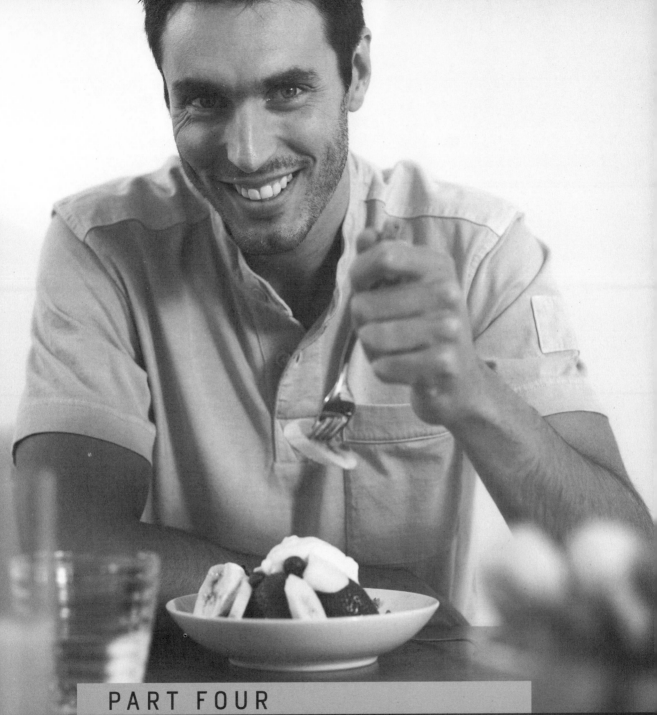

MAXIMUM IMMUNITY

YOUR IMMUNE SYSTEM IS YOUR BODY'S FIRST
AND LAST LINE OF DEFENSE AGAINST SOME VERY
BAD ENEMIES. FORTIFY YOUR INTERNAL SENTRIES
WITH THIS EIGHT-POINT PLAN

BY JEFF O'CONNELL

You might wonder why a professor of immunology would deliberately place behind his desk a bottle filled with a swirling elixir that lists among its ingredients echinacea, the supposedly immune-boosting wonder tonic. It sits there to illustrate a point. "The human immune system is extraordinarily robust, meaning it isn't easy to push off base," says Andrew Saxon, MD, who specializes in clinical immunology and allergy at UCLA. "But once it is thrown off base, beware of simple fixes." If a potion that a pimpled clerk in a convenience store rings up along with your Powerball ticket and beef jerky could really fend off a microorganism, the bugs that cause colds would be history by now.

Fad cures will fail, but your factory-installed immune system goes all the way back to the Model T versions of Homo sapiens. And in the intervening millennia, evolutionary fine-tuning produced impressive victories over everything from bubonic plague (a bacterial disease) to the Great Influenza of 1918 (a viral disease). Alas, these were fleeting leads in a race that won't end, short of human extinction—and even something as pesky as a common cold has left us in a dead heat today.

"Every time we make a move, the viruses, pathogens, and bacteria think of a countermove," says Hidde Ploegh, PhD, a professor of biology at MIT. "And there are some nasty customers in every category."

Indeed. Few are nastier than HIV, which causes an immunological pileup by disarming the very system needed to brake its advance. So, in addition to everything else mentioned below, cover your joystick with a condom before having sex. (But you already knew that.) To keep your immune system fully operational outside of the bedroom—with a tune-up and a power boost for good measure—make sure you can answer in the affirmative the eight questions that follow. Once you can, the bugs will start cruising around in search of easier competition, and you can perform at top speed.

ARE YOU TAKING IN ENOUGH CALORIES TO REPEL THE INVADERS?

WHY IT'S IMPORTANT: It takes calories to form antibodies and dispatch them to the front lines when germs invade. When your calorie intake dwindles, your body's priorities become keeping your heart beating and your lungs pumping—the functions needed to survive at that instant—while your immune system is left to operate at a deficit.

THE TEST: "To see if you're consuming enough calories, monitor your body weight (without clothes) on the scale in the morning," says nutritionist Christopher R. Mohr, PhD, RD, owner of Mohr Results. "Unless you're on a weight-loss program, your body weight shouldn't move more than a pound or two in either direction in a given week."

THE SOLUTION: "If you're losing weight, slowly add some healthy foods, such as fruits, vegetables, and mixed nuts," says Mohr. "If you're gaining, cut back a bit on your portions. Don't skip meals." Either way, dietary variety is vital. In fact, researchers at Colorado State University recently found that even if your consumption of fruits and vegetables is limited, you can boost the health benefits. The easiest way: Make sure there are always at least five different colors of produce in your supermarket shopping cart.

IS YOUR IMMUNE SYSTEM RESTED ENOUGH TO GO ALL OUT?

WHY IT'S IMPORTANT: Insufficient sleep depresses the immune system, opening the door to colds, upper-respiratory infections, and other nagging ills. You don't have to be wearing an orange jumpsuit and bedding down in Guantánamo, either: A study in *Psychosomatic Medicine* found that even minor sleep disturbances caused a significant drop in the number of cells whose job is to kill invaders.

THE TEST: Take the following self-test, "Do You Sleep Enough?", to see if you're getting enough shut-eye. Nodding off during the test is an automatic F.

THE SOLUTION: Consider your caffeine intake. If it's excessive, it might be not only screwing with your sleep patterns but also sabotaging your immune system. Studies show that caffeine suppresses the functions of key immune agents, such as lymphocytes and T cells. So what's considered "excessive" caffeine? Researchers in Ireland recently concluded that consuming more than 4 cups of regular coffee a day is probably enough to give your immune system an unwelcome jolt.

ARE YOUR BUG-KILLER CELLS FUELED UP AND READY TO ATTACK?

WHY IT'S IMPORTANT: Your immune cells treat an amino acid called glutamine as if it's high-test, and sometimes their tanks need topping off. "Glutamine comes from protein foods, and if you're not eating enough of those, your body will borrow from skeletal muscle, especially if you're working out," says Jose Antonio, PhD, CSCS, and CEO of the International Society of Sports Nutrition. In one study, marathon runners who took glutamine instead of a placebo had less chance of experiencing an upper-respiratory infection after racing.

THE TEST: Are you working out regularly? If so, keep it up—but down some glutamine.

THE SOLUTION: After exercising, try taking 5 to 15 grams of GNC Pro Performance L-Glutamine. Your white blood cells will thank you. And, for that matter, so will your muscles. When German researchers analyzed a series of muscle biopsies, they discovered that levels of glutamine

(continued on page 110)

>>DO YOU SLEEP ENOUGH?

1. How many hours of sleep do you average each night?

    A. 8 hours or more

    B. Around 6 to 7 hours

    C. 5 hours or less

Subtract an hour and 24 minutes from that total, because people confuse time spent in bed with time asleep, according to a study in the *American Journal of Epidemiology*. Researchers found that although the study participants averaged 7.5 hours in bed, only 6.1 of those hours were spent asleep. "People don't think they sleep enough, and they get even less sleep than they think," says study author Diane Lauderdale, PhD.

2. You hit your alarm clock's snooze button . . .

    A. At least once a morning

    B. Once or twice each week

    C. Once in a blue moon

If you're sleeping a full night and still reaching for the snooze, you could be suffering from sleep apnea, says Gerard Lombardo, MD, director of the Sleep Disorders Center at New York Methodist Hospital. It's a breathing disorder with symptoms ranging from snoring to stoppages in breathing throughout the night. Telltale signs: a neck size greater than 17 inches, recurring violent dreams, or gasping for air while asleep (reported by a bedmate).

3. Your last blood-pressure reading registered . . .

    A. Below 120 (systolic)/80 (diastolic) millimeters of mercury (mm Hg)

    B. From 120 to 139 mm Hg for systolic or 80 to 89 mm Hg for diastolic

    C. 140/90 mm Hg or higher

When Swedish researchers analyzed employees of a computer company, those with disturbed sleep patterns averaged 11 points higher in systolic and 9 points higher in diastolic blood pressure. One reason: Their levels of the stress hormone cortisol, a known BP booster, also increased.

4. Sex: How's your performance?

    A. I've been underperforming

    B. I've been over-performing

    C. I've only been doing solos

    D. I've performed like I always have

Just 2 hours of sleep deprivation impairs your erection-powering hormone levels by at least 40 percent, according to National Institutes of Health researchers. Your body needs sleep to fire the testosterone pumps full blast.

5. Your bedmate is . . .

A. A sound sleeper

B. A struggling sleeper

C. A major-league snorer

D. I sleep alone

"Sharing a bed with someone who has sleep problems can wreak havoc on your own sleep," says Bruce Corser, MD, medical director of the Sleep Management Institute in Cincinnati. According to a Harris poll of more than 1,300 adults who share a bed with a spouse or partner, one in four reports that their bedmate's sleep habits interfere with their own. Half of those people lose at least 3 hours of sleep a week.

6. You're eating dinner. If your stomach could speak, what would it say?

A. "Keep feeding me. I'm always hungry."

B. "Don't make me bigger. Eat right."

C. "This meal's good, but get me junk food!"

Two key hormones help regulate appetite: ghrelin and leptin. The former increases feelings of hunger; the latter suppresses appetite. People deprived of just 2 hours of sleep have 15 percent more ghrelin and 15 percent less leptin, according to researchers at England's University of Bristol.

Score your sleep

1. A = +2, B = -1, C = -2
2. A = -1, B = 0, C = +2
3. A = +2, B = 0, C = -1

4. A = -1, B = +2, C = 0, D = +1
5. A = +2, B = -1, C = -1, D = 0
6. A = -1, B = +2, C = -1

Up to 3 points: You need help before your sleep debt bankrupts your health. Two pro-sleep strategies: First, buy a TiVo. A survey by the National Sleep Foundation found that half of adults borrow from sleep to watch television. Second, try going to bed and getting up at the same times every day, even on the weekends. Sticking to a schedule helps reinforce your body's sleep-wake cycle and will help you sleep better at night.

4–8 points: You're spending enough time asleep to be aware of the benefits of getting more. Remember that occasional naps can repay sleep debt very efficiently.

9–12 points: Your healthy glow is blinding us.

—DAVID SCHIPPER

decreased as the donor's age increased, suggesting that supplementing with the amino acid now may help slow the steady muscle loss that usually occurs along with aging.

DOES YOUR BODY HAVE WHAT IT NEEDS TO REPAIR ITSELF AFTER EXERCISE?

WHY IT'S IMPORTANT: Working out does wonders for your body, but it sends free radicals scurrying around to clean up all that cellular debris. That's also an immune function, so you need to make sure your system has all it needs to stay strong on its other flanks: fighting bacteria and viruses. And the key to this? What you swallow after you sweat. In addition to boosting performance, postworkout nutrition helped stave off illness among Marine recruits in boot camp, according to a study in the *Journal of Applied Physiology*.

   THE TEST: If some or all of the following apply, you're not sleeping enough, eating enough, or both, for the amount of training you're doing.

» You're exhausted most of the time, but you
   have trouble sleeping at night.

» You're achy all over.

» You're getting weaker in the gym.

» You're injuring yourself (sprains, pulled muscles, and so on)
   frequently in small ways at the gym.

   THE SOLUTION: Your workouts have worn down your immune system. Along with dialing back the frequency and duration of your training sessions, the quickest, easiest, cheapest solution is drinking 17 ounces of chocolate milk as soon as you put that last dumbbell back on the weight rack. A study published recently in the *International Journal of Sports Nutrition and Exercise Metabolism* found that it was more effective as a form of postworkout nutrition than Endurox, a popular recovery drink.

DO YOU HAVE THE STOMACH FOR A STRONG IMMUNE SYSTEM?

WHY IT'S IMPORTANT: A chronically inflamed gut ultimately may play a role in everything from heart disease and cancer to auto-immune disorders—the unfortunate consequences of the immune system running amok and launching unprovoked attacks against healthy tissues. "When you're constantly in a heightened state of immune-function alert, it can have negative consequences for the whole body," says Susan M. Kleiner, PhD, RD, author of *The Power Food Nutrition Plan*.

PERCENTAGE OF EMPLOYEES WHO FREQUENTLY SHOW UP FOR WORK WHEN THEY ARE FEELING ILL: 80

THE TEST: Often feel a burning sensation in your stomach? You have either a bad habanero habit or, more likely, an infection.

THE SOLUTION: Mohr recommends eating a daily helping of one of the yogurts made by Stonyfield Farm. Its offerings help lay down healthy bacteria in the GI tract. And if you do happen to get sick—hospital-stay sick—don't stop spooning down the yogurt. When you go inpatient, you're at risk of being infected by the bacteria *Clostridium difficile*, which, as its Latin name suggests, is tough to beat. But while antibiotics are often useless, yogurt—specifically the bacteria *L. acidophilus*—is an antidote.

ARE YOUR IMMUNE ARMIES PATROLLING ALL THE PORTS OF ENTRY?

WHY IT'S IMPORTANT: Most of these tips focus on strengthening the host organism (that would be you) and its internal capacity to fight off microorganisms, rather than on the bugs themselves. But you should still keep your mouth, eyes, nose, ears, and other entry points hard to penetrate. Whatever you do, avoid using your own fingers to force bugs into those openings. Don't forget about your skin, either. It's no coincidence that burn victims often die of infection, or that eczema leads to recurring staph infections.

THE TEST: Check your skin for scabs. Think they're healthy, or at least macho? Think of them instead as crack houses for wayward bacteria. "A scab is a bacterial-culture medium," says Dr. Saxon. "With no blood supplying it, the scab cannot be healed by your immune system."

THE SOLUTION: "A scrape should always receive antibiotic ointment and a bandage and be cleaned up until you have nice pink, healthy tissue," says Dr. Saxon. "That's what we do to people in the hospital." Here's another skin tip: Don't shake a hand and make a friend if that person has a cold, or you may get one in return. Sounds obvious, but Dr. Saxon sees immunologists at conferences failing to take heed. If you shake a bugged hand by mistake, immediately wash your hands with semisoft natural soap. (Perfumed ones can irritate and actually provoke an immune response, while antibacterial soaps can lead to resistant bacteria over time.) Keep your fingernails trimmed short, too, and dig them into the bar while washing—most of the pathogens congregate around the nails. Also, your cuticles are designed specifically to keep bacteria out of your body, so if you're in the habit of using them as a snack, opt for a handful of nuts instead.

▶▶HOT-ROD YOUR GRANDMA'S CHICKEN SOUP

If she made chicken soup our way, its status as a cold and flu buster wouldn't just be urban legend. "The variety of nutrients in this chicken soup will ensure that your immune system is in tip-top shape," says its mastermind, Christopher R. Mohr, PhD, RD. Garlic and onions, for example, have powerful antibacterial and antiviral abilities. Even better, the added broth from the chicken provides some of the necessary fluids for your body.

1 tablespoon olive oil
1 clove garlic, sliced
½ red onion, sliced
2 cans (14 ounces each) low-sodium chicken broth
2 carrots, chopped
2 stalks celery, chopped
½ package frozen spinach
1 rotisserie chicken, cooked, boned, and shredded
Black pepper

Put the olive oil in a pot and heat over medium. Add the garlic and onion and sauté them until golden brown. Add the broth, carrots, and celery and cook until the vegetables become tender. Add the spinach and chicken and heat through. Season to taste with the pepper.

ARE YOU KEEPING YOUR SENTRIES SUPPLIED WITH ENOUGH WATER?

WHY IT'S IMPORTANT: Even overnight, during what amounts to an 8-hour fast, your immune reserves are being drained. Hydration becomes even more important when you're sick. Fluids not only transport nutrients to the illness site, but also take toxins away for disposal.

THE TEST: Check the color of your urine the first time you pee upon waking. Dark yellow? You need more water at night.

THE SOLUTION: When you wake up, drink water to replenish all the systems that have been active during the night. "Green, black, or white (not herbal) tea is another immune-friendly vehicle for consuming water," says Mohr. He also suggests Tropicana Pure Premium Immunity Defense orange juice. The added zinc and vitamin C won't prevent a cold, but they might decrease the severity and duration of symptoms.

> PERCENTAGE INCREASE IN THE EFFECTIVENESS OF THE FLU SHOT WHEN IT'S ADMINISTERED BEFORE NOVEMBER 12:
> **38**

DID YOU RECEIVE A FLU SHOT?

WHY IT'S IMPORTANT: To boost your immune system, rely on medical science as needed—like when it's time for a flu shot. "You're priming the immune system for when the real thing shows up by giving it a weakened form of some of the component parts of the virus you'll be exposed to upon infection," says Ploegh. "So it's already making antibodies and mounting the necessary cells to attack anything that might come in."

THE TEST: Shots aren't necessary for everybody, but if you have respiratory problems, heart problems, or asthma, for example, you definitely need protection from something as virulent as the flu.

THE SOLUTION: If you fall into any of these categories, get inoculated. If you don't, it's still not a bad idea to go for a shot every year or so, just to boost your immunity. The Centers for Disease Control and Prevention recommends October and November as the best months to get stuck, although studies show that after mid-November, the shots become less effective. Also, a study in the *Journal of the American Medical Association* found that the shots tend to work better when you're well rested.

FAST FOOD FIXES

STRESS, DEPRESSION, JOINT PAIN, POOR VISION,
AND MORE—FIX EVERYTHING WITH FOOD

BY PHILLIP RHODES

Consider this your age-defying, libido-lifting, cancer-beating, eyesight-saving, heart-strengthening, fat-fighting, decade-by-decade nutrition plan.

YOUR 20s: THE BEAT-STRESS DECADE

The average guy marries at 27. And although we're sure it's a coincidence, most episodes of major depression start around the same time. Perhaps the cause is a culmination of twentysomething stressors—the kind that come with 70-hour workweeks and late nights on the pub circuit.

But it's not just your mind that pays the price. A busy, high-stress lifestyle often leads to a diet of convenience—one that's lacking in vitamins and minerals, and overloaded with sugar, fat, and calories. The result: a body that never realizes its full potential.

See, this is the decade when your levels of muscle-building hormones—testosterone, DHEA, and growth hormone—hit their peak, making it the best time for you to pack on muscle. It's also your last chance to lay down new bone; by the time you're 30, your skeletal system is set. Poor nutrition not only inhibits your ability to do both, but also increases your risk of disease, weight gain, and mental breakdown—now, and for decades down the road.

But you can fight back with food; start today and you'll build a body that will last a lifetime.

The Problem: Undetected Depression

A Starbucks Chantico may boost your mood temporarily, but it won't improve your long-term outlook.

THE FIX: Eat 1 tablespoon of ground flaxseed daily. It's the best source of alpha-linolenic acid, or ALA—a healthy fat that improves the workings of the cerebral cortex, the area of the brain that processes sensory information, including that of pleasure, says Jean-Marie Bourre, PhD, a nutrition researcher at Hospital Fernand Widal in Paris. Find ground flaxseed online at www.drugstore.com or in the health-food section of your grocery store. To meet your quota, sprinkle it on salads, vegetables, and cereal, or mix it in a smoothie or shake.

> NUMBER OF PEOPLE WHO HAVE CALLED IN SICK BECAUSE OF STRESS RATHER THAN A PHYSICAL AILMENT:
> ## 4 in 10

The Problem: Cancer Is Incubating

Every hour, your body replicates 6 billion cells, creating copies of your DNA. But if you don't consume enough folate—a B vitamin that helps construct those cells—your body could produce irregular DNA, which can eventually cause cancer, says Ann Yelmokas McDermott, PhD, a nutrition scientist at Tufts University in Medford, Massachusetts. Trouble is, folate is hard to come by. The best natural food source is chicken liver, and few men get the folate their bodies require from fruits and vegetables.

THE FIX: Have a cup of folate-fortified cereal 4 days a week. Choose a brand—such as Total Raisin Bran or MultiGrain Cheerios—that provides at least 400 micrograms of folate per serving. Then top it with ½ cup of blackberries, raspberries, or strawberries. Berries aren't just a good nonliver source of folate; they're packed with antioxidants, which help thwart cancer by neutralizing DNA-damaging free radicals. They also offer a fringe benefit. Fructose—the sugar found in fruits and berries—can help you recover from another twentysomething problem: hangovers. That's because it speeds the rate at which your body metabolizes alcohol by up to 25 percent.

The Problem: No Time to Eat Healthy

A recent study at the University of California at Berkeley found that nearly one-third of the average guy's diet is pure junk—foods that provide no nutritive value, just calories.

THE FIX: Try vegetable-and-lean-meat combination meals, such as Birds Eye Voila! and Stouffer's Lean Cuisine Skillets; each takes just 10 to 15 minutes to go from freezer to plate. Eat an entire bag as a single portion (about 600 calories) and you've found the easiest way to down three full servings of vitamin-packed vegetables. Bonus: Harvard scientists found that every one-serving increase in daily vegetable intake decreases your risk of heart disease by 4 percent.

The Problem: Fast-Food Addiction

In a study published in the *Journal of the American College of Nutrition*, researchers discovered that men consume 1,000 calories each time they visit a fast-food restaurant. And, on average, men eat 500 more total calories on the days they drive-thru instead of drive past. Indulge just twice a week and that's 15 pounds of extra weight in a year.

THE FIX: Limit yourself to one "single" burger or sandwich, and make it the only food item you order. (Choose water, diet soda, or unsweetened tea or coffee as your beverage.) This damage-control strategy ensures that you won't overeat. For instance, if you use this approach at McDonald's, the fewest calories you'll down is a filling 260; the most is a manageable 730. And even an occasional Big Mac falls in between, at 560 calories.

The Problem: Untapped Muscles

Your twenties are your brawn-building years. But to maximize muscle growth, you need the right raw materials.

THE FIX: Beef. It's the perfect muscle food because it's packed with protein, zinc, and creatine. Down a hefty portion of each with this taco-salad recipe from *Men's Health* cover model and "Muscle Chow" columnist Gregg Avedon: Brown ½ pound of extra-lean ground beef over medium heat. As it cooks, sprinkle it with black pepper, 2 teaspoons of chili powder, and a couple dashes of Tabasco. Place the cooked beef, one diced tomato, and 2 tablespoons of low-fat cheese over a bed of lettuce, and top with salsa.

The Problem: You're Becoming More Injury Prone

Bones are a lot like reclusive coworkers; until one snaps, you aren't likely to give them much thought.

THE FIX: Drink two 8-ounce glasses of vitamin D–fortified low-fat milk every day. This provides your body with 600 milligrams of calcium and 5 micrograms of vitamin D, the perfect combination of nutrients to build break-resistant bones. Plus, in a 20-year study, U.K. researchers determined that men who drink more than 6 ounces of milk a day have half the risk of stroke of men who drink less.

YOUR 30s: THE MELT-FAT DECADE

The metabolic rate that allowed you to burn through super-size burritos in your twenties is slowing—dropping by 1 percent every 4 years. And even if the number on your scale isn't rising, it's likely you're getting fatter. In a study published in the *American Journal of Clinical Nutrition*, scientists found that men who managed to maintain their weight for 40 years still gained 3 pounds of fat each decade—while losing 3 pounds of muscle.

The likely reason: After you pass 30, your testosterone levels decrease by up to 1 percent a year. This means it becomes harder for you to build—or even maintain—metabolism-boosting muscle. (See the connection?) Another side effect: By 40, more than half of men develop some degree of erectile dysfunction.

But sagging testosterone levels aren't your only health hazard. Starting at age 30, your systolic blood pressure rises 4 points per decade, and joint degeneration begins to occur.

Here's how to turn back your biological clock—and keep midlife years in front of you.

The Problem: Corroding Joints

Even though arthritis doesn't usually set in until your fifties, the damage that causes it is happening now.

THE FIX: Eat three 6-ounce servings of cold-water fish weekly. Specifically, have salmon, mackerel, trout, halibut, or white tuna—each packs more than 1,000 milligrams of fish oil. A U.K. study found that regularly consuming this amount of fish oil appeared to halt cartilage-eating enzymes in 86 percent of people who are facing joint-replacement surgery. Fish oil slows down cartilage degeneration and reduces factors that cause inflammation, says lead researcher Bruce Caterson, PhD.

The Problem: Rising Blood Pressure

Some men are always close to their boiling points. And new research from the Netherlands may explain why. The scientists discovered that besides the obvious factors—obesity, lack of physical activity, and high salt consumption—diets containing too little potassium were the primary cause of hypertension. In their analysis, the scientists used 3,500 milligrams daily as the cutoff for defining a low potassium intake. The average intake for a man in his thirties? Only 3,100 milligrams.

THE FIX: Add ½ cup of beans, a banana, or a handful of raisins to your daily diet. Each will increase your potassium intake by about 400 milligrams a day, boosting you above that 3,500-milligram benchmark.

The Problem: Waning Sex Drive

Don't wither away down under.

THE FIX: Munch on two handfuls of walnuts, peanuts, or almonds every day. Research shows that men with diets high in monounsaturated fat—the kind found in nuts—have higher testosterone levels than those who don't eat enough of the healthy fat. Nuts are also the best food source of arginine, an amino acid that improves bloodflow throughout your body—including below the belt.

The Problem: Your Metabolism Is Slowing

By snacking on the right foods—those that are low in sugar but rich in protein—you'll keep your metabolic furnace stoked, and be less likely to binge between meals.

THE FIX: Have one slice of hard or semihard cheese—for instance, Cheddar, Swiss, or provolone—two or three times a day. Cheese has 7 grams of protein per slice and contains no sugar. That means it doesn't raise blood-sugar levels, so your body stays in fat-burning mode. Want an alternative? Opt for a cup of low-fat plain yogurt or a stick of beef jerky, or multitask with a handful of almonds. (See "Waning Sex Drive," above.)

The Problem: You Can't Lift as Much Weight

As testosterone levels start to drop, it takes longer for your muscles to return to full strength after each workout.

THE FIX: Eat broccoli and bell peppers. Together, they're packed with vitamins C and E, two nutrients that fight free radicals—rogue molecules that slow the repair of exercise-induced muscle damage, impeding recovery. Try this 15-minute meal from Avedon. It's infused with the most effective ingredients for speeding muscle recovery after a hard workout—vitamins C and E, high-quality protein, and slow-digesting carbohydrates. In a deep saucepan, sauté 1 tablespoon of chopped onion, ¼ of a red bell pepper (cut into long, thin strips), and a pinch of black pepper on medium heat for 2 minutes. Next, add ½ pound of turkey-breast strips and 1 teaspoon of sage. Brown the turkey for 2 minutes, then add 1 cup of chicken broth and 1 cup of broccoli florets. Bring to a boil for 1 minute, then stir in ½ cup of plain, uncooked couscous. Cover the pan, remove it from the heat, and let it sit for 5 to 10 minutes before serving.

The Problem: Every Lunch Is a Business Lunch

Dining out means restaurant megaportions—and, most likely, a mega-gut.

THE FIX: Trade that grilled-chicken sandwich for a grilled-chicken salad. U.K. researchers found that men who ate a low-glycemic lunch—one without bread, rice, or pasta—burned more fat for 3 hours after eating than those who ate a high-glycemic meal, even though both groups consumed the same number of calories. More smart choices: chicken stir-fry, fajitas sans the tortillas, or even a 6- to 8-ounce steak with a side salad or steamed vegetables.

YOUR 40s: THE FIGHT-DISEASE DECADE

Baldness, wrinkles, and back hair are the least of your worries; your body may be a walking time bomb. That's because approximately 30 percent of men in their forties have asymptomatic prostate cancer, according to research from the Barbara Ann Karmanos Cancer Institute. That is, the cancer is there but nearly undetectable. It's a terrifying prospect, but a reality in your forties, which might be labeled "the decade of disease."

The reason: Until age 44, accidents are the most likely cause of death in men. But once you reach 45, heart disease becomes your number-one threat, killing 36,000 fortysomething men every year.

And scientists at the University of California at Irvine discovered that men over 40 were up to twice as likely to develop melanomas than were women of the same age.

There's also an elevated risk of nonfatal diseases, such as macular degeneration, the leading cause of blindness. And don't forget about obesity: Even if you managed to sidestep it during your thirties, keeping your waistline in check doesn't become any easier as you get older.

The solution? A preemptive attack on your body's natural enemies. Your weapons: a knife and fork.

The Problem: A Fat Expense Account

Eating on the company is a fast way to inflate your gut.

THE FIX: Adopt a point system. Assign these values to menu items: 2 points for a salad; 3 points for an appetizer; 2 points for an entrée; 4 points for a dessert; and 2 points for an alcoholic beverage. Order whatever you want, but limit yourself to a total of 6 points. To follow this system, choose from a category only once.

The Problem: Cancer-Prone Skin

Mutating moles are scary, but food can help: National Cancer Institute researchers determined that people with the highest intakes of carotenoids—pigments that occur naturally in plants—were as much as six times less likely to develop skin cancer than those with the lowest intakes. "Beta-carotene is an internal sun protector," says Regina Goralczyk, PhD. That's because the vitamin plants itself in your skin, where its imperceptible orange and yellow pigments help deflect sunlight.

THE FIX: As a preventive, eat two sweet potatoes every week. This will provide you with the same amount of weekly beta-carotene as in men who demonstrated the lowest skin-cancer risk. Other top sources are carrots and cantaloupe.

The Problem: Shrinking Muscles

The average guy loses 6 pounds of muscle by the time he's 50. But, in addition to lifting weights, you can protect your hard-earned muscles by feeding them a steady supply of high-quality protein.

THE FIX: Tuna. Ounce for ounce, it's one of the best sources of protein—and contains zero saturated fat. To grill your way to a better body, follow this muscle-building recipe from Gregg Avedon. Brush a 6-ounce tuna steak with olive oil, lightly season it with freshly ground pepper, and place it on a grill preheated to medium. Grill until medium-rare to medium, for 7 to 10 minutes on each side. Meanwhile, mix 3 tablespoons of peanut butter, 1 tablespoon of lemon juice, 1 tablespoon of balsamic vinegar, 1 teaspoon of brown sugar, and 2 tablespoons of water in a bowl, and microwave the ingredients for 30 seconds. When the tuna is ready to eat, drizzle a small amount of the warm sauce on top. For a perfect complement, pair the tuna with ½ cup of wild rice.

The Problem: You're a Workaholic

Don't let long days at your desk undermine your healthy eating habits.

THE FIX: Order an inexpensive minifridge and have it shipped directly to your office. (We like the GE Spacemaker Compact Refrigerator; $130 at www.homedepot.com.) Stock it with food you won't be ashamed to carry into a meeting: pints of milk; individual packets of string cheese; a few ounces of turkey; and a couple of in-case-of-emergency microwave meals, such as Healthy Choice, Smart Ones, and South Beach brands.

The Problem: Elevated Risk of Prostate Cancer

Sex probably won't kill you, but your sex gland can. Fortunately, Harvard researchers found that men with the highest levels of selenium had a 48 percent lower incidence of advanced prostate cancer than those with the lowest intakes.

THE FIX: Eat three Brazil nuts every day. That'll provide you with 200 micrograms of selenium, the exact amount you need to keep your prostate-cancer risk at rock-bottom levels. Mushrooms help, too: A half cup of the cooked fungi—specifically, brown and portobello—contains more than 35 micrograms, or nearly 20 percent of the amount you need daily.

The Problem: Worsening Vision

You were first warned about going blind as a teen; this time, the threat is real. Thankfully, the National Institutes of Health found that people who consume the most lutein—a carotenoid found in plant foods—are 43 percent less likely to develop macular degeneration. Lutein helps filter blue light, preventing it from damaging retinal tissues.

THE FIX: Eat two servings of greens each day. Consider one serving to be ½ cup of cooked spinach, broccoli, or brussels sprouts.

The Problem: Narrowing Arteries

High cholesterol is a killer.

THE FIX: Grab a handful of grapes every day. Antioxidants in the skin of red grapes have been linked to lowering LDL cholesterol and preventing clogged arteries. A glass of red wine is also beneficial. In a recent Spanish study, scientists found that red wine reduced markers of arterial inflammation by 21 percent. Alcohol also thins your blood, just as a daily aspirin does.

INFECTION PROTECTION

BEAT SEVEN HIDDEN BIOHAZARDS THAT WANT
TO TAKE YOU DOWN

BY JENNIFER EVERETT

Even if avian flu never enters America, it's already in our heads. See, we checked with the Centers for Disease Control and Prevention, and as of right now, the only verifiable pandemic is fear. But that's the thing with bugs, whether they're cutting-board bacteria or ultravirulent viruses: They are the ultimate invisible enemy, often infecting us with anxiety before they've triggered a single immune response.

The key to staying safe—and sane—in a world crawling with germs is knowing which ones are worth worrying about. Ol' H5N1? Not unless you like your chicken so fresh that you raise your own. Bubonic plague? Only if you reside in New Mexico and play with prairie dogs. On the other hand, do you own a cell phone? Take a shower every day? If so, then we have some high-priority pathogens we'd like you to meet—and, with our help, defeat.

THE CELL PHONE

WHAT'S LURKING: Methicillin-resistant *Staphylococcus aureus* (MRSA)

Think of MRSA as staph on steroids; it's resistant to most antibiotics and can be deadly if it enters the bloodstream. And even though MRSA usually hides in hospitals, at least 12 percent of the infections in 2005 occurred in the general community, often inside locker rooms. Another hot zone: cell phones. When University of Arizona researchers tested 25 cell phones, 20 percent came up positive for MRSA. "When was the last time you cleaned your cell phone? I'm willing to bet never," says Charles Gerba, PhD, the study's lead researcher and coauthor of *The Germ Freak's Guide to Outwitting Cold and Flu*. "These things are very germy, especially the keypads and mouthpieces." Picture it:

Every time you dial a number or send a text message, you're transferring the germs on your hands to your phone and then straight to your mouth.

HOW TO BEAT IT: Sanitize your cell once a week with Clorox disinfecting wipes (or any of the supermarket-brand clones). "The wipes won't get into the internal parts of the phone and damage it the way a spray might," says Gerba. If you want more peace of mind, consider Motorola's new i870 cell phone ($300 with a 2-year Nextel contract). The i870 comes treated with AgION Antimicrobial, a very fine ceramic powder coating that contains silver ions, the same substance that's woven into some gym apparel to help inhibit the growth of bacteria.

THE SHOWER

WHAT'S LURKING: Methylobacter and Sphingomonas

Germs thrive in warm, wet environments, which is why they like showering with you. When Norman Pace, PhD, a professor of molecular biology at the University of Colorado at Boulder, tested five plastic shower curtains—including his own—he discovered millions of microbes lining every square inch, with 80 percent being either Methylobacter or Sphingomonas. What makes this finding worrisome is that studies of indoor pools show that both bugs can form an aerosol and rise into the air. "There's no doubt the same phenomenon occurs in the shower, and thus we're breathing in these potentially harmful bacteria," says Pace, though exactly how harmful is unclear. "We know people get sick for reasons we can't put our finger on. This could be one of them."

HOW TO BEAT THEM: You could hold your breath while you lather up, or you could simply make your shower less inviting for infectious agents. For starters, pull the curtain all the way closed after you're finished. This will help prevent bacteria from thriving inside the plastic folds. Or, better yet, opt for a fabric shower curtain and an all-metal showerhead. "These types of organisms feed on the organic compounds that form on plastic," says Pace. They also like to gorge on skin cells and other organic material that sloughs off in the shower, so if you go with a cloth curtain, toss it in the washing machine once a month, using the hottest water the fabric can handle.

HOSPITALS

WHAT'S LURKING: *Clostridium difficile*

Also known as *C. diff,* this bacteria has been causing diarrhea in hospitals for decades. Ironically, the bug remains dormant inside healthy people until they begin popping certain antibiotics, which eliminate beneficial bacteria that keep *C. diff* in check. But, as bad as it is to have the runs while relegated to a bedpan, there's a greater danger: Last winter, two studies in the *New England Journal of Medicine* identified a more virulent variation of *C. diff.* In an accompanying editorial, John G. Bartlett, MD, chief of infectious diseases at Johns Hopkins University, notes that "this *C. difficile* strain produces 16 to 23 times more toxins."

HOW TO BEAT IT: If you're going to be laid up in the hospital for more than a day, make sure your menu includes yogurt that contains "live" or "active" cultures. You'll be ingesting *L. acidophilus,* one of those good bacteria that can beat *C. diff* but is killed off by antibiotics. "It's an amazing thing. The number of cases of *C. diff* has dropped dramatically since we started serving yogurt," says Jimmy McDaniel, MD, a staff physician at Baxter Regional Medical Center in Arkansas. "Take a teaspoon morning, noon, and night, just as you would regular medicine." Try our favorite brand of live-culture yogurt: Stonyfield Farms Organic Nonfat, laced with *L. acidophilus* and several other microbial MVPs.

AIRPLANES

WHAT'S LURKING: Norovirus

Most cruises are all-you-can-eat . . . and all-you-can-expel, if Norovirus is on board. What most travelers don't realize, however, is that this bug can also hijack airplanes. A recent CDC study of a flight from London to Philadelphia shows that 9 percent of the passengers and more than half of the crew were stricken with diarrhea and/or vomiting within 18 to 60 hours of the flight. That norovirus could infect so many in so short a time doesn't surprise Mark Gendreau, MD, an emergency-medicine specialist who studies aircraft infectious disease for the Lahey Clinic in Burlington, Massachusetts. "When we look at how contagious a disease is, we calculate how many microorganisms of that species are required—from less than one to 100,000—to produce an infection," he explains. "Norovirus has a dose of 0.6, which means a single bacterium can produce a very serious outbreak."

HOW TO BEAT IT: Assume that the flight attendants are infected. Because they interact with everyone on the plane—and on any other flights they've been on that day—the attendants are the most likely people to contract and transmit norovirus. So if they hand you a beverage, drink it with a straw. And if they serve you a prepackaged meal, sanitize your hands after opening it. Not packing Purell? Soap and water is fine, but avoid whichever restroom the flight attendants are using.

Of course, you could escape norovirus only to catch a cold, especially if someone's hacking in your airspace. Dr. Gendreau's defense: "Typically, I'll turn the gasper [the overhead air vent] on at the lowest setting possible and aim it straight down so I don't feel the current," he says. "This circulates clean air without drawing germs toward you."

>>TOP 10 DIRTIEST PLACES

From 1999 to 2003, researchers gathered 1,061 surface samples and analyzed them for the presence of the following bio markers: alpha-amylase (indicating mucus, saliva, sweat, and urine), hemoglobin (blood marker), and urea (urine marker).

Surface: percent tested positive
for alpha-amylase, hemoglobin, or urea

Playground equipment: 44%

Bus armrests and rails: 35%

Public restroom surfaces: 25%

Shopping cart handles: 21%

Chair armrests: 21%

Escalator handrails: 19%

Customer-shared pens: 16%

Vending machine buttons: 14%

Public phones: 13%

Elevator buttons: 10%

GOLF COURSES

WHAT'S LURKING: West Nile virus

The water hazard at your golf course is also a West Nile hazard; it's where mosquitoes that carry the virus buzz around and breed. And while West Nile fever typically affects older, immune-compromised individuals, a newly identified condition called West Nile poliomyelitis can hit healthy adults in their 30s and 40s. "It's a very serious neuroinvasive disease that attacks the cells in the spinal cord that are responsible for motor strength and activity," says Taylor Harrison, MD, a professor of neurology at Emory University. "Some people regain movement of their limbs; others don't recover as well."

HOW TO BEAT IT: Simple: Steer clear of the drink. Also, "if the course is wet, it's a good idea to stay off the golf-cart path," says Gilbert Waldbauer, PhD, a professor emeritus of entomology at the University of Illinois and the author of *A Walk around the Pond: Insects in and over the Water.* "The puddles that form in the tracks are filled with stagnant water where larvae develop." He also suggests a midmorning tee time: "They're out in full force at dusk and dawn." To further shield yourself from skeeters, wear Buzz Off pants and shirts, apparel that's been treated with an EPA-approved insect repellent called permethrin. Both Tommy Hilfiger Golf (www.golfsmith.com) and Oxford Golf (www.oxfordgolf. com) make Buzz Off duds for duffers.

THE BEDROOM

WHAT'S LURKING: Chlamydia trachomatis

Chlamydia is the stealth STD—a woman can carry the bacteria without symptoms for several years, which means your partner could pass it on to you, even if you're currently monogamous. And once a guy gets chlamydia, he's at risk of developing nongonococcal urethritis (NGU), a bacterial infection of the urethra, says H. Hunter Handsfield, MD, a clinical professor of medicine at the University of Washington Center for AIDS and STD. NGU is one of the most common reasons men find themselves sitting in an STD clinic. Or standing, since NGU may cause dull testicular pain as well as cloudy discharge and frequent, painful urination. Left untreated, it can lead to infertility.

HOW TO BEAT IT: Either commit to wearing condoms or ask that your wife or girlfriend be tested for chlamydia. If you opt for the latter, tell her you'll be tested, too; it's possible for someone who's been cured of chlamydia to be reinfected by their partner. Think you may already have NGU? See your doctor—and take this article along.

≫A NEW RISK IN IRAQ

If insurgents don't get our soldiers, infections just might

Even though improvised explosive devices still pose the greatest danger to U.S. troops in Iraq, another hidden threat is festering under their feet: *Acinetobacter baumannii*, a strain of antibiotic-resistant bacteria that occasionally pops up in American hospitals but thrives in Iraqi soil. Since the start of the war, at least 300 U.S. soldiers have been infected with the bug, which can lead to brain damage, coma, or death.

"*Acinetobacter baumannii* is very dangerous to wounded soldiers or people who are weakened by an illness," says Col. Bruno Petruccelli, MD, director of epidemiology and disease surveillance for the U.S. Army Center for Health Promotion & Preventive Medicine. "If a resistant strain enters the bloodstream through an open wound, it can cause a prolonged infection." From there, the bacteria can travel to the lungs and central nervous system.

Most recently, a study from Walter Reed Army Medical Center found that 15 percent of wounded soldiers who returned stateside tested positive for *A. baumannii*. What's more, the bacteria's resistance to treatment is growing: Roughly 20 percent of cases in the United States are currently resistant to most antibiotics, up from 7 percent 3 years ago. "The frightening thing is, with the huge cost of drug development, there are very few new treatments on the horizon," says Lisa Maragakis, MD, an assistant professor in the division of infectious diseases at Johns Hopkins medical school.

Faced with this reality, some researchers have decided to get creative. Cornell University scientists, for example, recently discovered that combining three existing antibiotics killed all lab samples of *A. baumannii*. "Drug combinations may be our best weapon once the bacteria take hold," says Dr. Maragakis. "But vigilant decontamination and isolation are also vital to preventing more infections."

—COLLEEN CRONE

"Although NGU is very common, not all doctors are as insightful about it as they could be," says Dr. Handsfield, explaining that you'll often get faster results at an STD clinic. "Most men with NGU will be diagnosed and given a prescription on the spot." Antibiotics such as azithromycin and tetracycline have been shown to be effective 90 percent of the time.

CRAZY CURES

TRY THESE SIX STRANGE YET TOTALLY EFFECTIVE
SOLUTIONS TO YOUR MOST COMMON AILMENTS

BY LISA JONES

If you believe Johanna Brandt, she discovered a cure for cancer roughly 80 years ago while living in South Africa. The remedy: grapes. Bunches of them. In fact, all you can eat, because, well, grapes are all you can eat for 1 to 2 weeks, if you follow the plan outlined in Brandt's 1928 book *The Grape Cure*. Proof? She claims to have conquered her stomach cancer with the power of purple.

Needless to say, the medical establishment never swallowed grapes as the answer to cancer. And yet, as extreme—and potentially dangerous—as Brandt's prescription may be, today's researchers are uncovering compelling evidence that natural chemicals in the fruit of *Vitis vinifera* could help prevent and, yes, even treat certain types of tumors in mice. Granted, you wouldn't want to stake your life on a rodent in remission, but there are other examples of modern science finding that some really odd antidotes might be just crazy enough to work.

Bad back? Plug in your headphones. Bad breath? Screw in a lightbulb. These are two of the six strange-but-true treatments that we went from Australia to Israel to Ohio to gather. We aren't promising that any of them will cure cancer, but they are guaranteed to be completely seedless.

TREAT SLEEP APNEA WITH A DIDGERIDOO

"A didgeri-what?" you ask. While aborigines in Australia have been playing this long wooden trumpet for centuries, it's just recently been redefined as a modern-day medical device. Researchers reporting in the *British Medical Journal* evaluated 25 people with sleep apnea—a breath-stealing condition caused by flabby throat muscles—and found that those who took 4 months of didgeridoo (DIH-jeh-ree-doo) lessons had about 3½ times less daytime sleepiness than the folks who didn't blow their own horns. The newly minted musicians also snored significantly less. Credit vibrations that exercise tissue in the mouth and throat, says researcher Milo Puhan, PhD. "When these muscles are strengthened, the tongue has less tendency to obstruct the airway."

MAKE IT WORK FOR YOU: If huffing on a wooden tube to treat your sleep apnea sounds a tad too weird, then you probably aren't familiar with the alternatives. The most commonly prescribed option is continuous positive airway pressure (CPAP), which involves spending every night hooked up to a machine that pumps air down your throat to keep it from collapsing. The other approach is surgery, and that's only 30 to 60 percent effective. Now are you ready to toot the didgeridoo? You can pick up a beginner-friendly model for about $80 at L.A. Outback (www.laoutback.com). And don't worry; it's intuitive to learn, says co-owner Barry Martin. You purse your lips and blow into it with the beat.

QUIT SMOKING WITH TEXT MESSAGES

Any time you want a Marlboro, reach for your Motorola instead. Researchers at the University of Auckland in New Zealand compared how well two groups of smokers were doing in their attempts to quit. They discovered that those who received daily text messages containing tips on beating cravings plus motivational words from other quitters were twice as likely to kick ash as the people who went textless. What's more, rates of quitting for the cell-supported group remained high after 6 months. "People tend to carry their phones with them at all times, so it's a readily accessible means of providing cessation assistance," says study author Robyn Whittaker, MD. "It's also relatively anonymous and confidential."

MAKE IT WORK FOR YOU: When you're finally ready to stub your cigs, set a quit date and then go to www.backpackit.com, where you can write text messages to yourself and have them sent on preset days and times. Or, to prevent you from predicting every missive, you can use random delivery options, such as "later today" and "tomorrow morning." Either way, include words of encouragement and reminders about why you're quitting (such as a later exit from Earth). Next, go to your phone's message options and create a group list of your closest friends and family. Send a text message to all of them, asking that they shoot you encouragement on your quitting day and the days that follow. Save the messages you like and pull one up every time a craving strikes.

BEAT BACK PAIN WITH MUSIC

It's official: Brahms is the balm. Cleveland Clinic researchers recently found that when people with loused-up lumbar regions listened to music for 1 hour every day, they experienced a 20 percent reduction in back pain after just 1 week. "The effect may simply be due to music distracting your mind—or it could be that it induces muscle relaxation," says study author Sandra Siedlecki, PhD, RN. "New studies that examine the effect of music on stress hormones such as cortisol may shed more light."

MAKE IT WORK FOR YOU: Don't just flick on the radio and leave your relief to chance. In the study, those who chose their own tunes experienced significantly greater pain relief than the people given songs selected by the researchers. And it didn't matter if the self-styled DJs listened to heavy metal or light pop. "Different types of music had similar effects," says Siedlecki. So make a mix of your desert-island favorites and press "play" when back pain hits. But keep the volume in check: Research shows that loud sounds—even the toe-tapping kind—can raise cortisol levels, possibly negating any benefit.

ZAP BAD BREATH WITH BLUE LIGHT

Researchers at Hebrew University Hadassah School of Dental Medicine experimented with ways to fix a malodorous mouth, including shining some light on the problem. In a study reported in the *Journal of Medical Microbiology*, the scientists exposed saliva samples to various wavelengths of light and then conducted a sniff test. The winner: blue light—by a nose.

"It induces the production of oxygen radicals, which are harmful to anaerobic bacteria, the producers of bad breath," says study author Nir Sterer, DMD, PhD.

MAKE IT WORK FOR YOU: Until researchers develop a safe, handheld blue-light device, you'll need to get creative. To that end, try replacing the lightbulbs over your bathroom sink with a set of GE Reveal bulbs ($4)—they give off the necessary bug-bashing rays. Then just complete your normal twice-a-day routine—floss, brush, scrape, gargle. Whatever light that manages to filter into your mouth may help your halitosis, and it won't hurt—unless you stand on your tiptoes and bare your teeth to the bulbs; prolonged, close-up exposure to blue light has the potential to harm sensitive gum tissue.

MEND MUSCLE WITH CHERRIES

Recover from hefting 200 pounds of iron by lifting 12 ounces of cherry juice. In an 8-day study of weight-training men, University of Vermont researchers discovered that those who imbibed a tall glass of a cherry-juice blend twice a day retained more strength (18 percent) and experienced faster pain relief (1 day sooner) than men who downed cherry-flavored Kool-Aid. A concentration of inflammation-fighting antioxidants inside cherries helps erase the ache, says Declan Connolly, PhD, the study author. "They minimize the microscopic muscle tears that occur during forceful contraction."

MAKE IT WORK FOR YOU: Normally, calorie considerations would argue for chewing your cherries instead of drinking them. Only problem is that you'd have to eat dozens of cherries to realize the anti-inflammatory effect of one glass of the juice, which Dr. Connolly points out is really all anyone should need to feel results. What is important, however, is the timing of your imbibing. "It's best to drink it after lifting or any time you do a higher-intensity workout," he says. Look for a brand made with "red tart cherries" but without added sugar, such as Organic Just Tart Cherry from R.W. Knudsen ($5), or CherryPharm ($2.50. www.cherrypharm.com).

FIX AN ENLARGED PROSTATE WITH BOTOX

Physiologically speaking, an expanding gland and frown lines have nothing in common, except that the former can cause the latter. But recent research in the *British Journal of Urology International* shows that when men with benign prostatic hyperplasia (BPH) were given Botox injections in their prostates, most experienced a 30 percent improvement in their symptoms, including a reduced urge to urinate and an easier time of things when they did. Botox is believed to help beat BPH by blocking key nerves that contribute to the prostate's runaway cell production. In addition, the effects of a single injection last for a year, says study author Michael Chancellor, MD, which is about three times the duration of Botox-corrected crow's-feet.

MAKE IT WORK FOR YOU: "Botox is a good option for younger men who don't want to take a pill or have surgery," says Dr. Chancellor, adding that both can cause side effects ranging from fatigue to erectile dysfunction. "And even though it's an off-label use, more and more doctors are being trained to do it." (Ask your urologist about prostate botulinum-toxin therapy.) Obviously, it's harder to hit a target below the belt than one on someone's face, which is why doctors use ultrasound to help guide needle into gland. "It sounds worse than it really is; you can be off playing golf the same afternoon," says Dr. Chancellor.

BRAIN PAIN BEATER

TURN THE TABLES AND MAKE YOUR HEAD BANGERS BAWL

BY SETH PORGES

If misery loves company, then headache sufferers can count a king and an emperor among their kind. Elvis Presley and Julius Caesar shared the despair of a throbbin' noggin long before computer screens, construction workers, and Slurpee-induced brain freezes made headaches commonplace. If you add it all up, the total U.S. headache-care tab comes to roughly $4.3 billion yearly.

These skull crushers come in a mind-numbing array, often leaving men in the dark as to the source of their particular brain pain. To make matters worse, guys often don't differentiate between minor pangs and serious maladies, and don't seek medical help when they actually need it. "Headaches can be a serious problem and need to be treated like one," says David Dodick, MD, a neurologist at the Mayo Clinic Arizona in Scottsdale. Knowing what kind of headache you're confronting is the first step on the road to beating their pain once and for all.

TENSION HEADACHES

WHO SUFFERS THEM: Almost everyone

HOW OFTEN THEY COME: Can be every day for weeks

WHAT THEY FEEL LIKE: The Rock's got you in a headlock—and he's squeezing.

WHAT'S HAPPENING: "The pain receptors that litter your brain stem are misinterpreting harmless stimuli, such as stress and muscle tension, as a reason to cause pain," says Frederick Freitag, DO, a board member of the National Headache Foundation.

BEST WAY TO PREVENT THEM: Drink more water. "If you don't drink enough water, eventually you'll develop a headache," says Susan M. Kleiner, PhD, RD, author of *The Powerfood Nutrition Plan*. (In contrast,

PERCENTAGE OF MEN WHO'LL ENDURE TENSION HEADACHES EVENTUALLY:

70

alcohol contains tyramine, an amino acid thought to dilate blood vessels and cause headaches, Dr. Freitag says.)

HOW TO TREAT THEM: Pop some pills. But start out slowly, because the quicker you escalate the antiheadache arms race, the more susceptible you'll be to "rebounds." "These occur when your brain stops producing pain-fighting chemicals after you take too many painkillers," says Merle Diamond, MD, associate director of the Diamond Headache Clinic in Chicago.

That's why, for the occasional headache, the old adage of aspirin or ibuprofen and rest may indeed be the best medicine. If that doesn't do the job, up the ante by adding a few more ingredients to create the perfect antiheadache recipe:

250 milligrams of aspirin. Better yet, drop it in Alka-Seltzer—the carbonation enhances absorption of the painkiller.

▶▶WHERE DANGER LURKS

So-called secondary headaches warn of other, often far more serious problems that can range from meningitis to brain cancer. Only about 3 percent of headaches fall under this heading, but here's what to look for:

No family history: Some primary headaches have a hereditary basis. If no one else in your family has ever had headaches like the ones you're experiencing, it may be a sign of something more worrisome, says David Dodick, MD.

Extra symptoms: Numbness, feelings of confusion, weakness, tingling, fevers, and night sweats could be telltales. And if a new headache type appears after you turn 50, it's probably a secondary headache, says Dr. Dodick.

Sex bombs: "If you suffer one during intercourse, it could signal an aneurysm, or a weakening in the wall of a blood vessel," says Frederick Freitag, DO. Smaller ones present little or no risk; larger ones can kill when they rupture.

Bottom line: Resist the urge to shake off your secondary headache as a mere annoyance. If it's a minor headache, the proper treatment can help make it a rare occurrence. If it's something worse, seeking medical attention could save your life.

200 milligrams acetaminophen (you may know it as Tylenol).

100 milligrams caffeine (the amount in about 1 cup of coffee). Caffeine regulates brain receptors that put a hold on the throbbing head pain.

Researchers at the University of Essen in Germany recently found that these ingredients are most effective when taken together. Luckily, Excedrin combines them for you.

BONUS TIP: "Wrapping a towel around your head squeezes dilated blood vessels, giving you some relief," says Yousef Mohammad, MD, an assistant professor of neurology at Ohio State University medical center.

SILVER LINING: These headaches end. Really.

MIGRAINE HEADACHES

WHO SUFFERS THEM: Somewhere around 6 percent of all men

HOW OFTEN THEY COME: Unpredictable

WHAT THEY FEEL LIKE: A spiked metronome is chipping away your skull.

WHAT'S HAPPENING: Migraine sufferers are cursed with a hyperactive nervous system. This causes neurons to shuttle around the brain like Richard Simmons on acid, which can lead to hallucinations known as auras, exhausting your brain. "The brain senses this, thinks something is wrong, and responds by pumping extra blood through its blood vessels," says Dr. Mohammad. These blood-filled vessels inflate, causing throbbing head pain.

BEST WAY TO PREVENT THEM: Stress makes migraines worse, which in turn creates more stress. The result: "Migraines beget migraines," Dr. Freitag says. "Twenty to 30 minutes of aerobic exercise per day seems to be the best way to fight this." But don't even think about exercising during an attack; it'll only make things (much) worse.

HOW TO TREAT THEM: Take a triptan. This class of prescription drugs, which includes Maxalt and Imitrex, blocks the transmission of pain signals from the trigeminal nerve to the brain. Supplements can also help. Magnesium restores normal electrical activity in the brain, cooling the migraine's jets. B vitamins help smooth out cellular processes that, when malfunctioning, stimulate an overactive brain. And patients who took 3 milligrams melatonin a night saw their migraine frequency drop in half, according to a study published in the journal *Neurology*.

NUMBER OF PEOPLE WHO WILL BE STRICKEN WITH CLUSTER HEADACHES:

1 in 250

BONUS TIP: New research shows that injections of the antiwrinkle neurotoxin Botox into the muscles surrounding the skull may help chronic migraine sufferers. In a recent study led by Dr. Freitag and funded by Botox maker Allergan, Botox injections caused migraine frequency to drop by almost a third.

SILVER LINING: A study recently published in the journal *Headache* reveals that one by-product of having a superexcitable nervous system is a sex drive 20 percent higher than other men's.

CLUSTER HEADACHES

WHO SUFFERS THEM: As many as one in 250 individuals—often men and the young

HOW OFTEN THEY COME: Usually one to three times a day over periods lasting several weeks to several months

WHAT THEY FEEL LIKE: "Like a white-hot poker is shoved through your eye and another one is shoved through your temple," says Thomas Mikel, a 34-year-old sufferer of these brain pains nicknamed "suicide headaches."

WHAT'S HAPPENING: Many neurologists believe the pain results from malfunctions in the part of your brain responsible for your biological clock. "That's why people tend to have cluster headaches at the same time each day," says Dr. Dodick.

HOW TO TREAT THEM: (1) Because the pain is intense, cluster headaches require speedy relief. An injection of a triptan, such as Imitrex, eases the pain in just 15 minutes. (2) Inhaling pure oxygen at the rate of 10 liters per minute for 15 minutes keeps vessel-inflating blood from flowing to the brain.

BONUS TIP: Avoid aromatherapy.

SILVER LINING: Cluster headaches are rare, afflicting less than 1 percent of men, although men are twice as likely as women to suffer their ill effects.

FEED A COLD

If cold viruses kept calendars, they'd mark November through March "The Sneezin' Season." So keep using hand sanitizer, and develop a yen for yogurt: Eating yogurt may cut—by half—your risk of catching a cold, say Swedish researchers. They gave 262 people either a supplement containing *Lactobacillus reuteri*—healthy bacteria added to some yogurts—or a placebo daily for 80 days. At the end of the experiment, those taking the supplement were 2.5 times less likely to catch a cold than people popping a placebo. "*L. reuteri* stops viruses from binding to tissue," says lead author Anders Zachrisson, PhD. You can find the beneficial bug in Stonyfield Farm yogurt—the only U.S. brand with *L. reuteri*—or supplements in the refrigerated section of health-food stores.

TRY A FISHY PRESCRIPTION

If you have aching joints, you may be able to skip the Advil. New research from the University of Pittsburgh suggests that the omega-3 fats found in fish oil reduce chronic pain as well as ibuprofen and other nonsteroidal anti-inflammatory drugs (NSAIDs) do. When neck- and back-pain sufferers replaced their daily NSAID with 1.2 grams of fish oil for 10 weeks, 60 percent reported feeling better. In fact, 59 percent stopped taking their prescription NSAIDs altogether. Credit the twin powers of EPA and DHA, the essential fatty acids in fish oil, which are converted into prostaglandins—compounds that fight inflammation.

Supplement sooner, rather than later. After age 30, your body's ability to turn omega-3 fats into prostaglandins—and pain relief—starts to diminish. (We like Nordic Naturals Ultimate Omega; $27 at www.nordic naturals.com.)

PRESS THE FLESH

There's no switch you can flip to turn off back pain, but there may be an "off" button. Acupressure is more effective than physical therapy at relieving back pain, according to a recent study in the *British Medical Journal*. After assigning 129 back-pain sufferers to six sessions of either acupressure or physical therapy, researchers determined that, while both treatments provided similar short-term pain relief, those given the finger had 89 percent less pain after 6 months than the people treated with physical therapy.

The secret? Acupressure may help ease the ache by increasing bloodflow to the affected area, releasing endorphins—the body's natural pain relievers—and relaxing tense muscle tissue. To find a qualified acupressurist in your town, go to www.nccaom.org and search for someone certified in Asian bodywork therapy.

CUT BACK ON CARBS, CUT BACK ON HEADACHES

Cutting back on carbs may relieve you of more than a few extra pounds. In a new study, researchers at Albert Einstein College of Medicine found that low-carbohydrate diets help reduce the frequency and severity of headaches in regular sufferers. "Half of those surveyed said they attained the same kind of relief from low-carb diets as they did from a migraine medication," says study author C.J. Segal-Isaacson, EdD, RD.

Although the scientists aren't sure why a low-carb prescription helps headaches, they speculate that some people may be more sensitive to carbohydrates and the allergens they contain—such as gluten, a wheat protein. Take note of when your headaches occur: Forty percent of the patients reported pain after eating starchy or sugary foods.

SCRUB UP

The average work desk harbors 400 times more bacteria than the average toilet seat. And the desks of some kinds of employees tend to be grimier than others, according to researchers at the University of Arizona. In a 6-week study of 90 offices (and 616 surfaces), the average accountant's desk was found to harbor the most dirt—upward of 12,600 different types of bacteria per square inch.

STOP YOUR SNEEZING

Until humans come with HEPA filters, popping pills is the best defense against allergies. And over-the-counter allergy pills are more effective than prescription drugs. University of Chicago researchers gave 58 allergy sufferers 240 milligrams of OTC pseudoephedrine or 10 milligrams of the prescription drug Singulair for 2 weeks. Both relieved itchy eyes and sneezing, but the OTC drug cleared congestion better.

"The OTC drug caused none of its known side effects, like anxiety and insomnia," says Fuad Baroody, MD, the lead author. To lower your risk of side effects, swallow pseudoephedrine in the morning. Note that in some states, even though no prescription is necessary to purchase pseudoephedrine, the medication is kept behind the pharmacy counter to prevent purchases of large quantities for the purpose of making illegal methamphetamine.

GET SWIFFERIN'

Cleaning under your bed can yield more than loose change and lost socks; it could produce healthier lungs. A new study reveals that people who don't dust may be at an increased risk of asthma. When researchers at the University of Iowa interviewed 831 families and then analyzed their homes, they determined that the people living in dusty conditions were twice as likely to suffer asthma symptoms as those who could ace the white-glove test. Researchers blame endotoxins, chemicals that are released by the bacteria in dust and can wreak havoc on the lungs.

Because most people spend 8 to 10 hours a day breathing the air in their bedrooms, these are the most crucial rooms to keep clean, says Peter S. Thorne, PhD, the lead study author. He recommends vacuuming weekly, preferably using a machine equipped with a HEPA filter.

KEEP YOUR JOINTS YOUNG

In a study of nearly 1,000 men and women, University of North Carolina scientists found that people with the highest blood levels of selenium are nearly half as likely to develop arthritis. One 3.5-ounce serving of tuna provides more than 55 micrograms of the mineral—the minimum amount you should take in daily.

START A PILLOW FIGHT

As if sleeping on a bed of dust mites weren't disgusting enough, it turns out our pillows may be teeming with fungi, reports a recent British study. When researchers tested a sample of 10 pillows that had been in use for anywhere from 1½ to 20 years, they detected more than 1 million fungal spores in each of them. Synthetic pillows were the worst, with as many as 16 species present.

"The covers on feather pillows have to keep the feathers in, so they block fungus better," says lead author Ashley Woodcock, PhD. If you like synthetic and you're allergic to mold—or simply don't want to bury your face in fungus— buy a pillow cover designed to block allergens.

PERCENTAGE OF MEN WHO EVER FEEL DEPRESSED: 86

TREAT RLS TO ALLEVIATE DEPRESSION

Feeling down even though life's looking up? The problem may be in your legs, not your head. Treating restless legs syndrome (RLS) may alleviate depression in some men, say University of Kentucky researchers. In a study of 1,500 adults with RLS—a neurological condition that causes involuntary leg movements at night—researchers learned that 34 percent of the men were depressed and 20 percent had anxiety. Both rates are higher than those of the general population. Poor sleep caused by RLS may create the mood changes.

"Exercising and drinking less caffeine may boost dopamine levels, which reduces RLS symptoms," says lead author Barbara Phillips, MD.

NEW, IMPROVED POTATO

Call it the couch potato's potato. A U.K. company has created a new spud that, on average, contains 26 percent fewer carbohydrates and 33 percent fewer calories than the regular kind. It's called the Vivaldi potato; look for it in US grocery stores in 2008 or 2009.

PEE-POWERED GADGETS

Scientists in Singapore have developed a 1.5-volt battery that gets its juice from urine. When mixed with magnesium and copper, urine can produce as much electricity as a AA battery. More work is needed before we start seeing pee-powered gadgets.

SUPERFOOD

A Canadian firm has developed a flavorless product called Salba that the company claims will make any food healthier. One tablespoon of the additive, made from a strain of wild mint, reportedly delivers 1.5 milligrams of omega-3 fatty acids, 2.5 grams of fiber, and six times the calcium of a tablespoon of milk. Tortilla chips and salsa made with

Salba, such as Salba Smart Organic Yellow Corn Tortilla Chips, are available in stores (www.salbasmart.com).

MAGIC MARKER

The same technology used to nab shoplifters may soon stop doctors from cutting into the wrong limb. Washington University scientists have invented an alarm that sounds if a patient exits pre-op without his or her wristband being swiped by a special pen. This reminds surgeons to mark incision sites with the patient's input.

INFECTION-FIGHTING SPONGES

Despite their reputation as kitchen petri dishes, some sponges grow germ killers. Scottish researchers found that a sponge made of polyurethane was the only place they could culture an antibiotic capable of clobbering methicillin-resistant *Staphylococcus aureus*. Their goal is to use the discovery to make a mass-produced medication.

PEER INTO YOUR FUTURE

FIVE DIAGNOSTIC TOOLS IN YOUR MIRROR

1. THE CLUE: YOUR INDEX FINGER

The condition: Aggression

The reason: The shorter your index finger relative to your ring finger, the hotter your temper is likely to be, according to a Canadian study. Researchers examined hockey players' hands and learned that men with aggressive tendencies had the largest digit differences. "The more testosterone a fetus is exposed to in the womb, the greater the difference in finger length and the more likely a man is to be aggressive," says lead study author Peter Hurd, PhD.

The fix: Add visualization to your morning routine. Imagine constructive reactions to the aggression triggers that could arise in the coming day, says anger-management specialist Steven Korner, PhD.

2. THE CLUE: BOWLEGS

The condition: Arthritis

The reason: Out-of-whack alignment places a greater proportion of your weight on your knees, resulting in added pressure that may break down the delicate cushioning between the bones. This may prove crippling over time. "It's like wheel alignment in your car. If something is off-kilter, it's going to wear on your body," says Nicholas A. DiNubile, MD, author of *FrameWork: Your 7-Step Program for Healthy Muscles, Bones, and Joints.*

The fix: Cut the fat. Losing 10 pounds can reduce your risk of knee arthritis by as much as 50 percent, says Dr. DiNubile. "Weight amplifies pressure. Five extra pounds feels like 50 to your knees."

3. THE CLUE: YOUR COMPLEXION

The condition: Heart disease

The reason: British researchers recently found that men who suffered from acne as teenagers were 33 percent less likely to die of heart disease than their spotless peers. Researchers think the high levels of testosterone that cause acne may also prevent plaque from building up inside arteries.

The fix: Get busy. Sex stimulates testosterone production, says Christopher Steidle, MD, author of *Testosterone: A User's Manual*. Knock boots twice a week to be safe (and happy).

4. THE CLUE: YOUR HEAD

The condition: Sleep apnea

The reason: "People with wide, short heads also have shorter airways, which are easier to obstruct," says Mark Hans, DDS, a professor of orthodontics at Case Western Reserve University in Cleveland, Ohio.

The fix: Spoon. "Obstructive sleep apnea occurs when tissue in your upper airway relaxes and blocks the flow of air," says Edward Grandi, executive director of the American Sleep Apnea Association. Rolling onto your right or left can cause that tissue to fall to the side, clearing the obstruction.

5. THE CLUE: YOUR HEIGHT

The condition: Prostate cancer

The reason: During childhood, men taller than 5'9" may have produced extra amounts of a hormone linked to prostate cancer, says Stephen Freedland, MD, an assistant professor of urology at Duke University. Tall men also may have eaten more as children, which has been linked to a higher risk of prostate cancer as well.

The fix: Snack on seeds. Dried sunflower seeds are full of both vitamin E and selenium, which, according to a study published in the *Journal of Nutrition,* can significantly cut your risk of prostate cancer.

Do I have to drink extra fluids when I'm sick?

Absolutely, says *Men's Health* urology advisor Larry Lipshultz, MD. Symptoms such as nausea, vomiting, and fever often cause dehydration. As a result, your body fluids thicken, leading to congestion and headaches, which make you feel even worse. Drinking lots of fluids breaks the cycle by increasing circulation, thinning congested body fluids, and speeding the recovery process.

Does it make a difference if I choose generic over brand-name drugs?

A big difference—you'll save money. "A brand-name medication is the same chemical entity as the generic medication," and both get the same FDA testing, says Nicole Peterson, PharmD, an assistant professor at St. Louis College of Pharmacy. "Brand names just cost more." To see if there's a generic version of your medication, search at www.rxlist.com.

Should the side-effect lists on medicines worry me?

Not really, but don't ignore them altogether. They're as much a CYA move by drug companies' lawyers as they are a warning. Drugmakers obviously want to minimize their liability, says Patrick Finley, PharmD, a professor of clinical pharmacy at the University of California at San Francisco. Labels, ads, and package inserts "list almost every side effect that occurred during clinical trials and postmarketing surveillance." Which is why cringe-inducing caveats (mental disorders?!) aren't likely to apply.

Still, knowing if your hives are related to your meds can help stave off a more severe reaction. Look over the FDA-approved sheet enclosed with your medication, which lists common and serious side effects. Common side effects, such as nausea, are most likely to occur when you first start taking a medication.

"The vast majority of the time, people will develop a tolerance, and the nausea will go away within a few days," Finley says. But if a rash or anything on the "serious" list crops up, stop taking the med and consult your physician. Sometimes a dosage adjustment (especially for skinny guys) is all that's needed.

Can I make my medicines work better, faster?

Maybe, but it's not worth the risk. A study in *Pharmacy Times* found that taking antidepressants or antiarrhythmics with grapefruit juice increases the amount of medication that enters your bloodstream. The same with statins. "Increase" sounds good, but it also means an increase in the risk of side effects and toxicity. "If the statin level goes too high, muscle damage and wasting can occur," says Joel Zive, RPh, PharmD, of the American Pharmacists Association. Researchers at the University of North Carolina found that an enzyme called furanocoumarin in grapefruit can mess with your intestines' ability to control drug absorption. Without it, overdose is a possibility. Other liquids to watch for are milk, caffeinated beverages, and alcohol, all of which can bind to medications and block absorption. Our advice: Always wash down your pills with water.

I went to bed fine. I woke up and my back was out. What's wrong?

Carefully replay the past 24 hours. Did you lift a box awkwardly? Pull weeds? The pain of a strained muscle may not emerge until the body has had a chance to cool down—for instance, after 8 hours of sleep. "Strain is the most common back problem," says Steven Ludwig, MD, chief of spine surgery and an associate professor of orthopedics at the University of Maryland medical center. "As many as 85 percent of all Americans will experience this problem in their lifetimes."

The pain will fade in a few days, as long as you don't retreat to the couch. In fact, don't sit in one position for more than 30 minutes, Dr.

PERCENTAGE OF MEN WHO HAVE EVER BEEN TO A THERAPIST:

28

Ludwig says. Walking and mild stretching will keep the muscle from tightening more. Ibuprofen (such as Advil or Motrin) will reduce pain and swelling. Your call-the-doc alarm: numbness, tingling, or pain down the legs. That could indicate that a nerve is being pinched or rubbed.

My friends tell me I have wild mood swings. Are they crazy, or am I?

Everyone's entitled to a kicking-and-screaming freak-out now and then, but if you have a rep for flipping out, you're not just "blowing off steam." Look at the context, intensity, and duration of your mood swings, because they can be related to depression, says Husseini Manji, MD, director of the mood- and anxiety-disorders program at the National Institute of Mental Health.

The best natural fixes: sweat and sleep. Exercise may increase brain-cell creation, counteracting the stress your brain cells suffer during a depression-related illness. And skip that 2 a.m. rerun of *Three's Company* and go to bed instead. By staying up, you might be activating certain stress-related neurotransmitter systems. If these self-help methods don't help you lighten up, it's probably time to see a doctor.

How can I shorten the duration of a cold sore?

"The most effective way is to take an oral antiherpes drug, such as Acyclovir, Famvir, or Valtrex, within the first 24 to 48 hours of symptoms," says Kathleen Welsh, MD, a dermatologist in San Francisco. The warning sign of an outbreak is usually an itching, burning, tingling sensation in or around your lips.

If the sore has already erupted and is beginning to scab, use an over-the-counter medication such as Abreva to help ease symptoms and reduce redness. "Cold sores typically last 7 to 10 days, so it all depends on how early you catch and treat it," says Dr. Welsh. Cold sores are caused by the herpes simplex 1 virus and don't pop up unless something triggers them—usually stress or overexposure to the sun. If you're prone to them, ask your doctor about taking Acyclovir daily to prevent flare-ups. Taking a lysine amino-acid supplement (between 500 and 1,000 milligrams daily) or eating lysine-rich foods—beans, meat, dairy products, and fish—may help prevent outbreaks, though studies are inconclusive.

Can food cause my canker sores?

Sure. Likely culprits are sharp or crunchy foods such as pretzels or chips. But allergies, especially to wheat or gluten, can cause canker sores. Keep a food journal to match foods to outbreaks. And be sure to take a daily multivitamin with B12 and folic acid to eliminate any nutritional deficiency. If outbreaks continue to occur, see your doctor. Canker sores can be a sign of an impaired immune system.

It seems as if I always have to pee. Is this serious?

Possibly. But try to eliminate more benign causes first, by reducing your intake of fluids and caffeine, which stimulate the bladder to contract. Repeated trips to the bathroom at night could be insomnia in disguise. If you can eliminate these causes, head for a urologist— it could be a bladder infection, an enlarged prostate, or kidney disease.

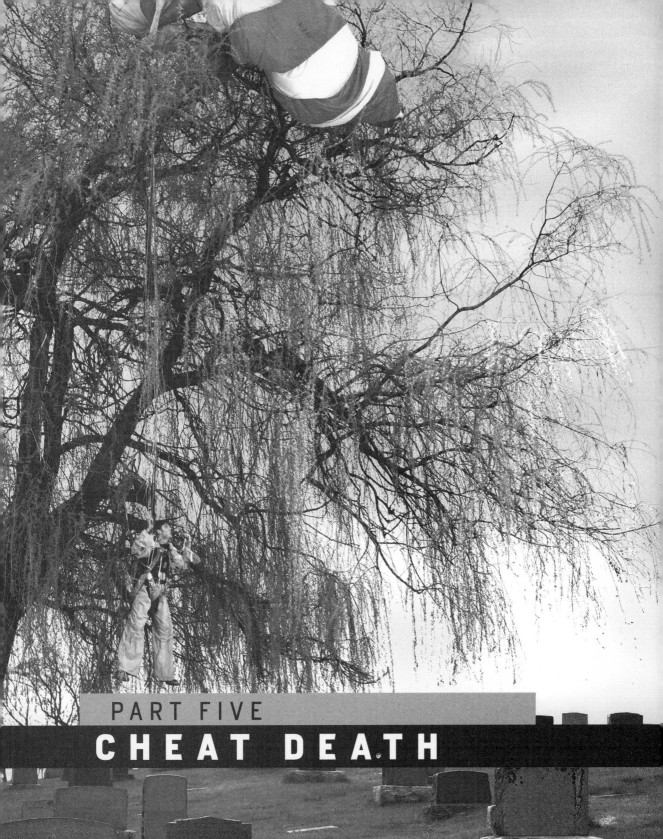

PART FIVE
CHEAT DEATH

YOUR WINNING NUMBERS

HIT THESE NUMBERS TO LEAVE DEATH IN THE DUST

BY TED SPIKER

What numbers are closest to your heart? Your child's birthday? Your wedding anniversary? Your one-rep-max bench press? All right, now we'll tell you which ones should be closest to your heart—and in a literal sense already are: LDL and HDL cholesterol, blood pressure, fasting glucose, C-reactive protein (CRP), and resting heart rate. Collectively, these are your vital signs. It's vital you know them, and if they aren't optimal, it's vital they improve—fast. And that brings us to another number: 5.

"I think a hell of a lot could change in 5 weeks," says David Katz, MD, an associate professor of public health at Yale University. "You could drop your blood pressure by 10 points. You could drop cholesterol as much as 20 percent." Same goes for the other life-and-death digits. In fact, start our plan on January 1, and come Valentine's Day, you'll hold a set of winning numbers you won't find on any lottery ticket.

GAUGE YOUR GAINS

Before you begin, have your blood pressure measured; request blood work, being sure to ask for a "high-sensitivity" CRP test; and buy a heart-rate monitor—we like the Polar F11 ($160). After 5 weeks, check your vitals again.

Vital Sign #1: Cholesterol

Whereas many doctors like to describe LDL cholesterol as "gunk," we found one who prefers a more incendiary image: "LDL represents the arsonists, and HDL represents the fire department," says Roger Blumenthal, MD, director of the Johns Hopkins Ciccarone Center for the Prevention of Heart Disease. "And a good fire department can usually prevent any long-lasting damage." Your goal: LDL lower than 130 milligrams per deciliter (mg/dl) and HDL higher than 40 mg/dl.

REINVENT BREAKFAST: Start your day with something besides razor burn. Instead, down an 8-ounce glass of juice that's half orange and half white grapefruit. The sour stuff is loaded with the flavonoid naringin, which Korean researchers found can lower LDL levels by as much as 17 percent. As for the OJ, it can boost HDL (by as much as 21 percent, if you drink three glasses daily). Next, mix crushed walnuts into yogurt or drop them on cereal; a new study in *Angiology* says that eating walnuts can raise HDL by 9 percent. Finally, swap your morning coffee for tea. USDA researchers found that drinking tea can cut LDL by 11 percent.

Vital Sign #2: Blood Pressure

Every hose has its bursting point, and your blood vessels are no different. But even if you avoid a messy blowout—i.e., a hemorrhagic stroke—hypertension can still level a hit. "It puts people at risk of heart attacks, heart failure, and kidney failure," says Paul Thompson, MD, a cardiologist at Hartford Hospital in Connecticut. Try to hold your BP below 120/80 millimeters of mercury (mmHg).

HANDLE LIFE'S HEADACHES: There may be no bigger pain in the cranium than a crazed work environment. To keep it from raising your BP, vent to your wife or girlfriend every evening; a new Canadian study shows that when work-stressed subjects received support from their partners, their systolic pressure dropped an average of 2.5 mmHg. After you're finished, take two aspirin. Spanish researchers recently

READ UP ON IT

found that hypertensive people who took 162 milligrams of aspirin before bed decreased their systolic pressure by 6.8 mmHg and their diastolic by 4.6 mmHg. (Check with your doctor first.) Last step before you sleep: Pray. New research shows that men who pray frequently have 3.5 percent lower diastolic BP than once-in-a-while worshipers.

Vital Sign #3: Resting Heart Rate

Your life isn't in your hands—it's in your heart. "Resting heart rate is one of the better predictors of longevity," says Dr. Thompson. In a study in the *New England Journal of Medicine*, men whose resting heart rates were above 75 beats per minute (bpm) were three times more likely to die of a heart attack than those with lower rates. Aim for 65 bpm.

KEEP YOUR TICKER GUESSING: "If you do cardio training at lower intensity and add higher intensity once or twice a week, your resting heart rate will drop," says Neal Henderson, CSCS, sports-science coordinator at the Boulder Center for Sports Medicine in Colorado. Train for a half hour at 60 to 80 percent of your maximum heart rate three times a week—but on 1 day, pick a random point and run (or bike) to it as fast as you can. Return at a slower pace, so it takes twice as long to get back to the start. Choose a new point, either nearer or farther, for your second sprint and make the return trip in the same manner as before. Repeat to fatigue. To do this on a treadmill, run at your fastest speed for 0.2 mile, then lower the speed by half and jog 0.2 mile. Repeat, alternating between 0.4, 0.3, 0.5, and 0.2 mile until you're tired.

Vital Sign #4: Fasting Glucose

Your fasting glucose level is your diabetes meter: As it rises, so does your risk of developing the disease. "Diabetes leads to devastating consequences—an elevated risk of heart disease, kidney disease, and eye damage," says Jonathan Samet, MD, a professor of medicine at Johns Hopkins. Worse, a study in the *Journal of the American Medical Association* shows that those with glucose levels over 140 mg/dl—40 mg/dl above normal—have a 29 percent higher risk of dying of cancer.

DEVELOP YOUR SENSITIVE SIDE: To lower your fasting glucose, you need to improve your body's ability to utilize blood sugar, a.k.a. your

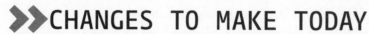

CHANGES TO MAKE TODAY

There's no time like the present for these simple fixes.

Hide your alarm clock: You won't be able to hit the snooze button. Research shows that people who sleep 7 hours a night live longer than those who log 8.

Brush and floss: The reduction in bacteria can cut your heart-attack and stroke risk. Bonus: better breath.

Take a walk: Daily. The extra time in the sun will increase your stores of vitamin D, which in turn may lower your odds of heart disease and prostate cancer.

insulin sensitivity. And the best way to do that is by losing weight—and lifting some. At the same time, supplement with conjugated linoleic acid (CLA). Canadian researchers noted that people who popped 4 grams of CLA daily had a 27 percent jump in insulin sensitivity after just 8 weeks. For an extra boost, replace 600 calories in your diet with a Hershey's Extra Dark chocolate bar; according to a new Italian study, this can quadruple insulin sensitivity in 2 weeks.

Vital Sign #5: C-Reactive Protein

Lower your CRP and you may never need CPR. That's because elevated CRP is often a sign of arterial inflammation—and heart disease. CRP is up there with cholesterol as a predictor of heart problems, says Barbara Nicklas, PhD, a professor of internal medicine at Wake Forest University in Winston-Salem, North Carolina. High CRP—over 1 milligram per liter—has also been linked to another man killer: prostate cancer.

NEUTRALIZE IT WITH NUTRIENTS: Swallow the tag-team treatment of vitamin C and magnesium. University of California at Berkeley researchers recently showed that taking a daily 500 milligrams of vitamin C supplement can decrease CRP levels by 24 percent. And according to a new study in the *Journal of the American College of Nutrition*, people low on magnesium are up to two times more likely to have elevated CRP levels than those meeting their quota. If you want a healthy dose of both nutrients, pick up GNC Men's Mega Men.

THE SKIN CANCER EPIDEMIC

MORE AMERICAN MEN WILL DEVELOP SKIN CANCER THIS YEAR THAN WILL GET PROSTATE, LUNG, OR COLON CANCER COMBINED. AND YOU COULD BE AMONG THE THOUSANDS WHO DIE. OPEN YOUR EYES

BY CHRISTOPHER MCDOUGALL

Take a good long look at yourself in the mirror. There's a good chance you're either a Chris Dale or a John Flanagan.

That means you're twentysomething and starting to get both hands around a real relationship and career—the Chris Dale scenario. Or you're pushing 40 with a little money under your belt, and a little flab over it—à la John Flanagan. You've had that sunspot, or birthmark, or whatever it is, for years, but it's never grown or even itched. How could you know that it's silently, painlessly ticking toward eruption?

You may escape death, depending on which description you fit. Still, death will leave a calling card: You'll have scars on your face, arms, and back, and a suspended sentence hanging over your head, because far more aggressive skin cancer could suddenly appear at any time for the rest of your life.

But you'll be the lucky one.

There are basically two types of skin cancer—lethal and disfiguring. The lethal kind is melanoma. It killed Bob Marley and Burgess Meredith, and might have killed Troy Aikman at the start of the 1998 NFL season and John McCain during the 2000 presidential campaign if they hadn't been saved by speedy surgery. Worldwide, one person will die of melanoma every hour, because the disease is fast and extremely aggressive: Once it penetrates your skin and enters your bloodstream, it can travel with nightmarish nimbleness, attacking your brain and every other organ in a matter of weeks.

Basal-cell and squamous-cell carcinomas, on the other hand, very rarely kill. They're the disfiguring type of skin cancer, munching away at your face and chest and arms like a flesh-eating virus. Left untreated for too long, they can cost you chunks of your ears, cheeks, chest, and arms. Nearly 1 million Americans have basal-cell carcinoma, and if you add in cases of squamous cell and melanoma, skin malignancies rank as the most common cancer in the United States.

They're also among the most predictable cancers, usually attacking older, fair-skinned people who've spent decades under blazing rays. Or at least that used to be the profile. Dermatologists have recently noticed that a rising number of their cancer patients are remarkably young. "It's becoming a regular occurrence: A 30-year-old has a red spot on his cheek that doesn't go away, and he can't believe what I have to tell him," says Roger Ceilley, MD, who has observed legions of suntanned teens and sunbaked farmers in his dual roles as a practicing specialist and clinical professor of dermatology at the University of Iowa. Another dermatologist in Boston, David Horne, MD, adds, "I recently treated an 18-year-old with skin cancer, which would have been unheard of 10, 20 years ago."

Last August, researchers at the Mayo Clinic confirmed in the lab what Dr. Ceilley and other dermatologists have been seeing in the field: Skin-cancer rates are shooting up among people under 40. According to the study, only 18 out of every 100,000 Americans under age 40 were diagnosed with basal-cell carcinoma in the 1970s; today, that rate has jumped to nearly 30 per 100,000. Squamous cell has become even more prevalent: It has quadrupled in the under-40 population. Formerly afflicting one in every 100,000 people, it now attacks four per 100,000.

This new battlefield in the war on cancer has emerged just when other key fronts are reporting progress. Leukemia, lung cancer, and colon cancer are all on the decline, thanks to medication, prevention, and early detection, but rates of melanoma—which should be the easiest cancer to prevent and detect—have nearly doubled over the past decade. The outbreaks have become so prevalent that the Skin Cancer Foundation estimates that within the next 5 years, one in every 50 Americans will have melanoma.

"These are truly frightening developments," says Randall K. Roenigk, MD, coauthor of the Mayo Clinic study and chairman of the department of dermatology at the clinic's college of medicine, in Rochester, Minnesota. "Something that is largely preventable not only has become epidemic, but also keeps on accelerating." Dr. Roenigk thought he'd lost the capacity for surprise by the time he'd finished compiling data for the study, but even he was startled when he recently found skin cancer gnawing at the nose of a patient—who was only 12 years old.

Unlike the mysterious origins of most diseases, tracing this epidemic back to its beginning is fairly simple: The seeds were sown 50 years ago, most likely in California, when suntans went from stigma to fashion statement. Before that, a ruddy bronze glow was mostly reserved for farmhands and stevedores. "It used to be associated with the lower classes, the laborers," says Dr. Horne. "Only in our lifetime have people begun lying in the sun to 'improve' their appearance—and now they're paying for it."

We could also be paying the price for abusing the environment as badly as we've abused our skin, Dr. Horne adds. "If the ozone layer is thinning as rapidly as some believe, then increased ultraviolet intensity would certainly be a factor," he says. "We haven't been measuring the UV index for very long, so it's impossible to say whether the increased cancer rates come from more exposure—more people spending more time in the sun—or a greenhouse effect, but it could be a combination of both."

But whether we're being punished for neglecting nature or ourselves, men are taking the brunt of the hit. You might think of female skin as being more delicate and consequently more vulnerable, but the truth is, men face a much higher skin-cancer risk than women. We're twice as likely to develop basal-cell or squamous-cell cancer and significantly more prone to melanoma (a one-in-58 chance, as opposed to one in 82 for women). Men are also more likely to die of melanoma, with an estimated 4,910 succumbing last year, compared with 2,860 women.

Breasts are the major reason men are more susceptible. Because guys don't have them, they spend more time shirtless in the sun. "Melanoma in men is most common on the upper back, where it can grow deep and thick," explains Diane Berson, MD, an assistant professor of dermatology at Cornell University's Weill Medical College. "That's not surprising, when you consider that from an early age, they're outside with their shirts off cutting the lawn, raking leaves, playing sports. They can have melanoma for a long time and think it's only a freckle."

Chris Dale's sister Amanda had seen that mole on his scalp for years, ever since Chris got his hair buzzed high and tight for the army. But it wasn't until the spring of 2004, after she'd taken a "skin-care essentials" class in her massage-therapy school, that she realized it could be more than a birthmark and began nagging him about seeing a dermatologist.

Chris must've told Amanda a million times that he couldn't afford a doctor's bill. He'd just been discharged from the military because of his bad knees, and at 24, he was still working only part-time for the sheriff's office and not yet eligible for health-care coverage.

Besides, the army docs had scoped him out from tip to toe when he was inducted the year before, and even more thoroughly when he was medically discharged 6 months later. He wasn't any big sun worshiper, either. Sure, he'd hung out at the beach—after all, he lived in St. Augustine, Florida, and spent a few childhood years in the US Virgin Islands, thanks to his dad's National Park Service job. But if he was spending a day in the sun, it was usually in a wool uniform. Chris had been a war buff since he was barely out of diapers, shooting his own black-powder musket by the time he was 5 and using his vacation time to attend Civil War reenactments. Besides, he snorted to his sister, he didn't even have a tan; his skin was as pale as his white T-shirt, and when he patrolled the beach on his sheriff's department ATV, he slathered on plenty of sunscreen.

"But Amanda, being a Scorpio and an older sister, had to have the last word," says Pattie Dale, Chris's mom. "She said she'd pay for it herself, and even make the appointment with her dermatologist." Chris grumbled his way to the doctor's office, and sure enough, it was just a benign birthmark. "Nothing to worry about," the doctor said.

But the next day, the doctor called back. He'd had the mole biopsied, just to be sure, and discovered he'd made a mistake. Chris had melanoma.

Meanwhile, up in New York City, John Flanagan was planning a getaway to the Hamptons. All you'd need is a glimpse of his blond Hollywood shag and wraparound midnight shades to guess that John would never miss winters in the Caribbean or summer weekends on an exclusive beach. Right before he left, though, he surrendered to his girlfriend's urging and went to have that little spot on his cheek checked out by a dermatologist.

At 40, and with a creamy, Irish-English complexion, John figured that an age spot or two was inevitable. He'd done his bit to stall time with high-end moisturizers, but he knew the years he'd spent in Los Angeles must have taken a toll on his skin. Back then, he rarely went to work without having spent at least an hour by the pool, just soaking in the warmth and thinking about his buddies shivering in the perpetual shadow of Manhattan high-rises.

Now that John was back in New York, he barely even saw the sun for weeks at a time. He made his living raising cash for film and real-estate projects, which meant lots of late-night networking in exclusive clubs and a workday that usually began when the sun was sinking. He'd gotten a bit of a burn at his weekend place in Woodstock, though, so he figured it made sense to check with a doctor about sunscreens before he hit the beach.

"Yes," the dermatologist agreed. "You'll need to get that spot scraped and biopsied."

Scraped? Guess again, doc. No way John was going to show up in the Hamptons with a gash on his face, looking like he'd been clawed in a bar fight. He'd deal with it as soon as he got back.

A single forgetful day can be all it takes to endanger your life, warns William Gallagher, PhD, the lead scientist of a groundbreaking new study examining why men are more likely than women to die of melanoma. If you neglect to smear on SPF one time, you're already at risk: One blistering sunburn in childhood can more than double your chances of developing the disease.

Last year, Dr. Gallagher's team at the UCD Conway Institute of Biomolecular and Biomedical Research in Dublin, began examining the DNA of cancer cells from a young man with melanoma. What they discovered was an association between aggressive melanoma and an odd mutation that exists only on a gene in the Y chromosome—which, of course, is present only in males. "It's a striking, very strange gene,"

Dr. Gallagher explains by phone from Ireland. "If the gene is turned off, you appear to have thick, aggressive melanoma tumors. If it's turned on, you tend to have thinner, nonaggressive melanomas."

The thicker the melanoma tumor, the slimmer your hopes of survival: Thickness is ranked on an escalating scale from Level 1 to Level 5, and the chances of beating even Level 3 or Level 4 melanoma are only about 10 percent.

"Men really have a double whammy, because another feature of more aggressive melanoma is drug resistance," Dr. Gallagher adds. "So not only is it spreading more rapidly, but it's also far more difficult to treat."

Dr. Gallagher's next challenge is finding out whether the gene is actually a trigger or just a red flag that goes up when the melanoma mechanism is activated. And if it is a trigger, as his evidence suggests, what role do the sun's rays play in tripping it? Is there a specific amount of ultraviolet light that can flip the switch?

Ultraviolet light has already been established as the prime mover in less-lethal forms of skin cancer. According to the Skin Cancer Foundation, more than 90 percent of all skin cancers are caused by sun exposure, while regular sun protection throughout childhood can reduce the risk of the disease by a staggering 80 percent. "Your DNA actually gets broken when sunlight hits the cell," says Dr. Roenigk. "That's all a suntan is—broken cells trying to rebuild themselves. But over time, the damaged cells get tired and don't rebuild themselves as well."

So, once again, technology rides to the rescue—tanning beds are the answer, right? "They're actually more dangerous," says David Goldberg, MD, a Manhattan-based dermatologist and vice president of the Skin Cancer Foundation. "They're terrible." One misconception is the notion that tanning beds are safer than natural light because they don't cause sunburns. "There are two types of UV light—A and B. Type B causes burns, but type A actually penetrates deeper and causes more long-term damage. And it's type A you find in tanning beds," Dr. Goldberg explains. "That is one industry that's long overdue for regulation."

If you're fair-skinned, you should actually be thankful for the burn warning UVB light provides. "Darker-complected men who don't burn think they're invincible," says Dr. Berson. True, they do have a natural advantage, since melanin—the pigment in our skin—helps screen the deeper layers of the epidermis. But your Sicilian granddad doesn't guarantee you unlimited nude-beach privileges: Just because your skin tans more gently doesn't mean it isn't being invisibly damaged.

"At least a lighter-skinned person gets the heads-up of a sunburn once in a while and takes precautions," says Dr. Berson. "But you'll find other men outside all the time with their shirts off, who could be slowly developing something that goes undetected until it's too late."

In July 2004, a few weeks after he learned he had Level 2 melanoma, Chris Dale submitted to the scalpel again. His dermatologist had previously removed the surface layers of his mole, but now that they knew it was malignant, a surgeon would cut deep into Chris's scalp and try to slice out every trace of the tumor before it spread.

"I'm going to beat this," Chris said, and he wasn't just being defiant. He was young, and the disease had been caught when it was only a few layers deep. Plus, Chris was taking all the right steps, no matter how painful. He was scheduled to begin training as a corrections officer that autumn, but he decided to start chemo right away, even though it meant he'd be nauseated and exhausted.

Chris injected the drugs at night, hoping to sleep off the effects, but he still had to stagger through many days at the academy. Somehow, he fought through; he became one of the top marksmen in his class and was appointed squad leader. And, come October 2004, he received an even better reward: A CT scan showed that his body was tumor-free. Thrilled, Chris and his fiancée, Mandy, began planning their wedding. They'd have it next fall, they decided, after he graduated from the corrections academy and began full-time work with the sheriff's office. "You never saw a guy with a bigger Howdy Doody grin," one of his instructors recalled.

About that time, up in New York, John Flanagan was making a second visit to his dermatologist. Again, the doctor insisted that John needed to have his sun spot analyzed, but there was something he just couldn't make the doctor understand: John always spent Christmas on St. Barts. Seriously, how could he go walking around one of the world's toniest island resorts with some thuggish-looking bandage on his face?

Besides, the spot didn't look any worse, so what was the hurry? He'd deal with it when he got back.

Luckily, a fantastic device that can detect early-stage skin cancer has already been invented. You've got one, in fact.

"Men look at themselves in the mirror every day when they shave," says Dr. Roenigk. "Don't they notice that spot on their face and wonder, Hey, where'd that come from? Of all the cancers, this is the only one you can actually see!"

And yet denial can be blinding. Dr. Roenigk once treated a man in his forties with a tumor nearly 9 inches long on his chest. The man came in only because his golf club banned him from the showers—he was bleeding all over the towels. What that golfer lacked in self-preservation and basic hygiene, he made up for in luck: The tumor was basal cell, not melanoma, so even though it had penetrated between his ribs, he survived.

▶▶IS IT A MOLE OR MELANOMA?

Make a date with a dermatologist if you scan your skin and see one of these trouble spots.

Basal-cell carcinoma: It's the most common form of skin cancer, affecting 800,000 Americans each year. In fact, it's the most common of all cancers.

Symptoms include a scarlike area with poorly defined borders and a shiny surface (this can indicate the presence of an aggressive tumor), a reddish patch or irritated area, or a pink growth with a slightly elevated border and a crusted indentation in the center.

Squamous-cell carcinoma: The second most common skin cancer, it afflicts more than 200,000 Americans each year. Symptoms include an open sore that bleeds and crusts over or a scaly red patch with an irregular border that crusts and bleeds.

Melanoma: The most serious form of skin cancer—deadly if left untreated. Symptoms include a small, even-colored bump that's symmetrical and often firm to the touch; or a flat or slightly raised discolored patch that has irregular borders and is somewhat geometrical in form. (You may see areas of tan, brown, black, red, blue, or white.)

Caught early enough, melanoma is a relatively easy cancer to control, because it can be attacked without having to open the skull or operate around delicate internal organs. But control isn't the same as a cure; surgery and chemotherapy can usually wipe out the tumors, but only temporarily. Melanoma is notoriously tenacious and a constant threat to reappear, so the best you can hope for is a tie, never outright victory.

Long-term solutions could be available within the next few years, but only on the precondition of early detection. Dr. Gallagher is experimenting with decitabine, a medication he believes may reactivate the non-aggressive-melanoma gene in men. "We're hoping to find a focused dosage that could be viewed as a prototype," he says. "In our experiments with mice, we've been able to dramatically reduce the size of the tumor and almost eradicate it."

A custom-made melanoma vaccine may also be on the way from the U.S.-based company Antigenics. Currently in late-stage testing, Oncophage is created from a patient's own melanoma tumor: Doctors extract a supply of "heat-shock proteins," a type of protein produced when cells are under extreme stress. Because heat-shock proteins contain antigens, injecting them back into the bloodstream signals the immune system to attack the tumor cells—and leave healthy cells alone. Oncophage isn't nearly powerful enough to destroy entire tumors, but it could be an antidote against recurrences. Once the melanoma has been surgically removed, the vaccine could help the immune system overwhelm new tumors before they have a chance to develop, says John Kirkwood, MD, the director of the melanoma center at the University of Pittsburgh Cancer Institute. "Men's ears should be perking up, because of their heightened risk."

Curiously, sunlight may also reduce melanoma's capacity to kill. According to researchers at Memorial Sloan-Kettering Cancer Center, a study of 528 patients with early-stage melanoma shows that those who'd had the most sun prior to diagnosis stood a better chance of survival. One plausible theory is that vitamin D, produced by exposure to the sun, helps slow the spread of cancer. Another possibility is that the sunlight breaks down collagen in the skin, turning it into a barrier that blocks the melanoma from penetrating into the blood or lymphatic system. But

(continued on page 170)

>>THE YOUNG MAN'S CANCER

We're developing colon cancer at record rates—and have the scars to prove it. Fight back with this tumor-proofing plan

Research from the University of California at Los Angeles shows that the incidence of colon cancer among men in their 20s and 30s has increased by 17 percent over the past 20 years, leading experts to theorize that this generation is paying for its sedentary, fast-food-filled childhood. Worse, the UCLA researchers also found that when young men develop the disease, they're more likely to have later-stage and higher-grade tumors. Meaning, if a twentysomething is diagnosed with colon cancer, his odds of surviving it might well have been worse than his grandfather's.

And that's why the best anticancer strategy is to prevent a tumor from taking hold in the first place. "The damage that is going to cause colon cancer, even when you're 50, may be happening right now," says Mark Welton, MD, a *Men's Health* advisor and chief of colorectal surgery at the Stanford Cancer Center. "There are ways to prevent it, so why not use them?" Here are six of these ways and how they can help you build a cast-iron colon.

Get berried alive: We don't usually recommend eating rat food, but in an Ohio State University study, rats that were fed raspberries and then injected with a chemical that causes colon cancer developed 80 percent fewer malignant tumors than did rodents without a berry to gnaw on. "Compounds in berries, such as anthocyanins and polyphenolics, inhibit blood-vessel formation, which is necessary to keep tumors growing," says lead researcher Gary Stoner, PhD, adding that "human trials are under way, and we presume the results will be similar."

Shop around for black raspberries, which have 40 percent more antioxidants than the red kind, according to lab tests. And when you get home, freeze 'em. Berries are about 90 percent water, so this will raise the concentration of the preventive substances, says Stoner. Wrap a bunch in a paper towel, then again in aluminum foil, and place them in the freezer. After a few hours, take the berries out, let them thaw, and dry them before eating.

Radiate good health: The sun may not shine there, but UV rays can still save your butt. That's because when sunlight hits any exposed skin, it stimulates the body's production of vitamin D—a shortage of which can lead to colon cancer. In an 8-year study from the University of California at San Diego, people with the lowest levels of D had double the risk of developing colon cancer, compared with those who had enough of the nutrient.

"Vitamin D alters the growth of colon cells to help prevent them from becoming malignant," says Michael Holick, MD, PhD, a professor of medicine at Boston University. If cold weather keeps you covered up, pop 1,000 IU of vitamin D3, a.k.a. cholecalciferol, the same type your body manufactures. In the warmer months, Dr. Holick recommends leaving your skin bare for 10 minutes before slathering on sunscreen; even an SPF of 8 reduces your ability to make vitamin D by 95 percent.

Turn up your training: Next time you hop on your bike or slip on your running shoes, pretend your life depends on the pace you set—because it does. University of Utah research shows that high-intensity cardiovascular exercise can cut your risk of colon cancer. Credit cardio's ability to lower insulin levels. Insulin may promote tumors by triggering cells to divide, says study author Mary Slattery, MD.

In her research, Dr. Slattery found that 40 minutes a day of vigorous exercise, such as running, lap swimming, cross-country skiing, or cycling, affords the most protection. Can't schedule that much sweat? Do what you can, but hit 65 percent of your maximum heart rate or higher—your bowels will still benefit. British researchers found that cardio work speeds up gut transit, the time it takes digested food to pass through the colon. And the faster food exits, the less time carcinogens are around to mutate healthy cells.

Nibble on some ears: Based on the visual evidence, you'd think that corn leaves your colon the way it went in: intact. But that isn't the microscopic reality. A University of Maryland lab study shows that inositol hexaphosphate (IP6), a component of fiber found abundantly in corn, prevents the growth of colon cancer. "IP6 causes cells to behave normally, putting them into a healthier state," says lead researcher A.K. Shamsuddin, MD, PhD. "Plus, it will actually cause cancerous cells to stop dividing."

Whether you eat it off the cob or out of the can, coat your corn with a little butter. Sure, you'll get some saturated fat, but you'll also ingest conjugated linoleic acid (CLA), a fat that can fight cancer, according to research from Stockholm's Karolinska Institute. "For every two servings of high-fat dairy foods eaten per day, the risk of colon cancer decreased by 34 percent," says study author Susanna Larsson, PhD. We say, stop at two.

Employ a curry-up offense: Indian food has an obvious downside—no medium-rare cow on the menu—and one lifesaving upside—the curry in darn near everything. Louisiana State University researchers recently found that when colon-cancer cells

(continued)

were exposed to curcumin—the yellow pigment that gives curry its color—25 percent were destroyed within a day.

"Studies have also shown that curcumin reduces the formation of blood vessels in cancerous cells and inhibits the cells' movement," says study author Anping Chen, PhD. Given all this, it's no wonder India has one of the lowest colon-cancer rates in the world. To grab some protection for yourself, order Indian at least once a week (any dish that has "curry" in the name) or top your chicken, vegetables, or rice with turmeric, a spice that has a high curcumin content.

And for dessert? Swallow a baby aspirin; research shows that the anti-cancer benefits of curcumin may increase in the presence of nonsteroidal anti-inflammatory drugs, such as aspirin.

White out your risk: Men with colon cancer have something in common with arthritic old people: COX-2 enzymes, a part of the inflammation response that can fuel arthritis and tumors. If a carcinogen such as, say, secondhand smoke enters your body and comes into contact with COX-2 enzymes, the cancer-causing agent will become even stronger. The solution, besides banning carcinogens from your body? Well, doctors give arthritis sufferers a script for a COX-2 inhibitor, but we're handing you a shopping list. "There are many COX-2 inhibitors in your refrigerator, such as fish, thanks to the omega-3 fatty acids, and white tea," says Mitch Gaynor, MD, an assistant clinical professor at Weill Medical College at Cornell University. In fact, new research from Oregon State University shows that, compared with green tea, the white kind has a greater ability to prevent DNA damage and inhibit cancer-cell activity. Drink a cup of Stash Exotica white tea (the brand used in the study) and swallow a packet of Coromega omega-3 supplement daily.

—DAVID SCHIPPER

whatever the explanation, it's still a painfully weak blessing: Better to avoid excess sun and never get cancer in the first place than hope a few more rays will blunt it.

"At this point, you can't hope to outguess melanoma and head it off at the pass," says Dr. Gallagher. "It may disappear and lie dormant for years, then reappear with frightening voraciousness. There are two things you can never underestimate about skin cancer: speed and unpredictability."

In May 2005, Chris and Mandy had to change their wedding plans.

He'd gone in for another CT scan, and the tumors that had vanished 9 months before had suddenly reappeared throughout his body. "It was bizarre," says Mandy. "He suddenly had lumps on top of lumps."

By the time the radiologists were finished counting, they'd discovered 70 tumors in Chris's abdomen, brain, lymph nodes . . . everywhere. He was immediately started on the most powerful barrage of chemotherapy his oncologist thought Chris could survive, including the newest and most aggressive protocol available, a regimen of high-dose interleukin-2. His family scrambled to put together a wedding for Chris and Mandy in 5 days; no matter what, the couple was determined to keep on living, and fighting.

Chris made it to his 25th birthday. On October 9, he was wheeled from the hospital to a surprise birthday party, where his friends and "family" from the sheriff's department turned out by the hundreds to wish him well and cheer him on. "I've got too much to live for," Chris told his kid brother, a soldier who'd rushed home from duty in South Korea to make the party. Two weeks later, Chris died.

"I still can't believe it," Mandy says. "To go from a mole to a funeral home—it's so strange. When I tell people what killed Chris, they go, 'A mole? How can a mole kill anyone?' They see all these ads and fundraisers for breast cancer and don't realize that it isn't nearly as lethal as skin cancer."

Somehow, John Flanagan got the break that Chris Dale couldn't find. The same month that Chris and Mandy were being married in a hasty, death-cheating wedding on the beach of St. Augustine, John was finally having a biopsy performed. The doctor found melanoma on his back and basal-cell carcinoma on his face and arm.

"I have an 8-inch scar on my back," John Flanagan tells me one afternoon in New York. He also has a bandage beneath his eye and another on his arm. "Every aspect of my life is changed," he says. It's not the scars that worry him; it's the loneliness of being an early prophet in a world that has yet to get the message about melanoma. "If I want to run or play tennis, or my girlfriend wants to go to the beach, what do I do?" John asks. "You know what America is like—we associate a tan with being healthy and successful. So I'm going to spend my life as the pasty-faced guy?"

He doesn't wait for an answer. "I know the alternative."

HEART SMARTS

TURN BACK THE CLOCK ON YOUR TICKER
WITH THESE FIVE SECRETS

BY ERIN HOBDAY

I was 11, sitting at our kitchen table with my dad and two sisters, when Dad's eyes suddenly rolled back in his head.

He slumped and fell clean off his chair, hitting the cold tile floor with a thud. The three of us jumped up, shrieking, and I dialed 911. Dad came to before the paramedics arrived, and he told us not to worry. "It was nothing," he said, and then made us swear not to tell Mom.

Flash forward 12 years. Dad, 51, is walking around a hospital room with two stents and a pacemaker in his chest, the calling cards of his heart attack. If he (and his doctor) had known back then what I know now, his heart muscle might not have suffered irreparable damage. Passing out, you see, is a sign of arrhythmia, a treatable condition that causes heart attacks, strokes, even sudden death.

Over the past few years, cardiologists across the country have begun aggressively trying to prevent heart disease in at-risk men, rather than treating them only after their blood pumps have broken down. "My patients who follow a preventive treatment program almost always live free of heart attacks," says Arthur Agatston, MD, author of *The South Beach Heart Program*. To help you spot subtle risk factors and correct them before they bury you, we canvassed cardiologists at leading research institutes to compile this list of things they wish you knew.

YOUR HEART'S MORTAL ENEMY
IS OFTEN INVISIBLE TO DOCTORS

"I was taught in medical school that when a heart attack happens, vessels have closed gradually, like pipes filling up with sludge," says Dr. Agatston. "We now know that blockages occur suddenly, from soft-plaque ruptures, which often go undetected by standard cholesterol tests and exercise stress tests." The soft plaques resemble pimples in the arterial walls, except instead of pus, they're filled with cholesterol.

WHY IT'S SO DANGEROUS: When those pimples pop, a small blood clot forms to heal the injury, followed by scar tissue and tiny calcifications along the arterial wall. By then, you're already incubating an attack, which strikes when a violent explosion of one of the pustules creates a clot big enough to block an artery.

HOW TO ID THE PROBLEM: If you have a family history of heart disease, schedule a 64-slice CT scan. It's the only test that snaps pictures of the heart quickly enough to reveal minute calcifications in the coronary arteries. Just make sure the scanner has ECG dose modulation, the latest radiation-limiting technology. If trouble's spotted, you may need statins.

HOW TO DEFEND YOURSELF: Toss pecans onto your salad or into your oatmeal. Loma Linda University researchers had 24 people replace 20 percent of their daily calories with pecans for a month, and found the nuts lowered levels of lipid oxidation (the process that turns cholesterol into plaque) by 7 percent, enough to help ward off arterial damage. "Pecans are rich in gamma-tocopherol, a form of vitamin E that isn't in supplements," says lead author Ella Haddad, DrPH, RD. Even a handful a day can help, she says.

AN UNTRAINED HEART WON'T REACH THE FINISH LINE

Not every heart test needs to take place in a cath lab. In a 23-year study of 6,000 men in the *New England Journal of Medicine*, researchers revealed that the greatest predictor of death from heart attack was the ability of a man's heart rate to adapt during and after a workout. "The faster your heart rate goes down after exercise, the healthier you are," says Steven Nissen, MD, chairman of cardiovascular medicine at the Cleveland Clinic.

WHY IT'S SO DANGEROUS: Those men whose heart rates didn't drop by at least 25 beats per minute (bpm) within 1 minute of finishing an intense workout were more likely to suffer a fatal heart attack than those whose heart rates dropped efficiently. The reason? How your heart

PERCENTAGE A SINGLE-SERVING INCREASE IN DAILY FRUIT OR VEGETABLE INTAKE REDUCES HEART DISEASE RISK:

4

adapts to exercise is a good indication of how well it will respond to the extreme stress produced before and during an actual infarction.

HOW TO ID THE PROBLEM: Complete 10 minutes of sprints, check your heart rate, and then check it again 1 minute later.

HOW TO DEFEND YOURSELF: Improve your heart-rate variability by applying the principles of interval training to your lifting regimen. Wear a heart-rate monitor and don't end your first set until the monitor reads 160 bpm, says Alan Stein, CSCS. "Then wait till it drops below 130 bpm to begin your next set."

YOU'VE NEVER EVEN HEARD OF THE CHOLESTEROL THAT WANTS YOU DEAD

Researchers now realize that the size of cholesterol particles is even more important than their number. Small particles of LDL, called LP(a), are a particularly damaging form of cholesterol, according to Michael Ozner, MD, medical director of the Cardiovascular Prevention Institute of South Florida. These particles aren't only smaller, they have a tail, says Dr. Ozner, making it easier for them to sneak into the arterial wall. On the flipside, the larger your HDL particles, the more easily they can usher LDL cholesterol out of your arteries.

WHY IT'S SO DANGEROUS: A recent study in the *Journal of the American College of Cardiology* reveals that people with high LP(a) were 10 times more likely to suffer a heart attack than those with lower levels.

HOW TO ID THE PROBLEM: Ask your doctor to schedule a Vertical Auto Profile (VAP) test. (Check it out at www.thevaptest.com. It's covered by most insurance plans.) This detailed blood profile includes a measure of LP(a)—an ideal level is below 10 milligrams per deciliter—as well as big and small HDL particles.

HOW TO DEFEND YOURSELF: Diet, exercise, and even statins have proven ineffective against LP(a). But in a review of 8 years of studies on prescription niacin, Dutch researchers determined that swallowing 2 grams of this potent B vitamin lowered LP(a) by 17 percent and raised the number of large HDL particles by 18 percent. Ask your doctor for a slow-release version of niacin. Research has shown that these formulations produce fewer side effects.

CARBOHYDRATES, NOT FAT, ARE THE REAL HEARTBREAKERS

The more carbohydrates you consume, the higher your blood sugar and, in turn, your levels of insulin, a hormone that lets us use sugar as energy. But excess insulin may also increase your risk of heart disease, according to a review in *Preventive Medicine*. "The inflammatory process leading to hardening of the arteries is mediated through insulin," says Wolfgang Kopp, MD, the study's lead author. Translation: High levels of insulin boost your body's production of stress hormones, which send blood pressure skyrocketing. That increased pressure damages the arterial wall, making it easier for cholesterol to slip inside.

WHY IT'S SO DANGEROUS: Insulin may not act alone. It's theorized that the excess carbohydrates that cause insulin to increase to an unhealthy level are turned into triglycerides in your liver. And the more triglycerides you have circulating in your bloodstream, the more LP(a)—the lethally small cholesterol—you're likely to have.

HOW TO ID THE PROBLEM: Johns Hopkins University researchers showed that for every 1 percent increase in hemoglobin A1c (HbA1c), an indicator of long-term blood-sugar levels, patients experienced a 14 percent increase in heart-disease risk. If diabetes appears anywhere on your family tree, schedule an HbA1c test. A level higher than 4.6 percent of total hemoglobin often warrants dietary changes and sometimes blood-sugar-lowering drugs.

HOW TO DEFEND YOURSELF: Pour yourself a cabernet. According to a recent study in the *Annals of Epidemiology*, small amounts of alcohol may help control your blood sugar, and, by extension, your insulin. Researchers studied the drinking habits of people with type-2 diabetes and found that compared with teetotalers, those who indulged in just one alcoholic beverage per night had levels of HbA1c that were 1.3 percentage points lower on average.

YOUR HEART MIGHT BE MISFIRING

One in four men will develop an irregular heartbeat, or arrhythmia, by the time they reach 40. Yet they often don't experience obvious symptoms until they're clutching their chests during cardiac arrest or they suffer a stroke. Your heartbeat originates in the sinoatrial (SA) node, a collection of specialized heart cells that acts as your heart's control center, says Jennifer Cummings, MD, director of electrophysiology research at the Cleveland Clinic. "It reacts to information from your body and brain about how much blood needs to be pumped, then sends an electrical impulse telling your heart when to beat."

▶▶RELAX—YOU'RE NOT DYING

Here are four alarming chest sensations that can impersonate an infarction.

A fluttering or pounding heartbeat: "Some perfectly healthy and normal individuals may feel extra or skipped heartbeats on occasion, and those can be benign," says P. K. Shah, MD, a *Men's Health* cardiology advisor. If the sensation is brief and the onset gradual, they are probably the harmless result of too much caffeine or stress. However, frequent flutterings, or those accompanied by lightheadedness or dizziness, could be serious.

Chest pressure when you swallow: If you feel a squeezing pain beneath your breastbone and it hurts to swallow, especially in the evening, you may just have heartburn or, at worst, an esophageal spasm. But if it persists most nights of the week, see your doctor to rule out gastroesophageal reflux disease or other more serious conditions.

Shooting pain on one side: "Sharp, fleeting pain on the left side of the chest is typically not life-threatening," says John Elefteriades, MD, a *Men's Health* cardiology advisor. It can signal pleurisy (an inflammation of the lung lining), a muscle pull, or even a broken bone.

Mild pressure, shortness of breath, and numbness: Hyperventilation is commonly mistaken for a heart attack. If the pressure in your chest isn't severe, and you lose feeling in your lips or hands, you may simply be hyperventilating. Lie down, try to relax, and breathe into a paper bag for 5 minutes. Still have symptoms? Call 911.

WHY IT'S SO DANGEROUS: "When an arrhythmia occurs, the heart stops listening to the SA node, turning its attention to other electrical signals," says Dr. Cummings. One form of arrhythmia, called atrial fibrillation, or AFib, can occur even in young athletic men. "It's like there are 300 voices inside the heart telling it what to do," says Dr. Cummings. Chaotic heartbeats cause the blood to swirl and eddy instead of flowing smoothly through the ventricles, and clots form as a result.

HOW TO ID THE PROBLEM: One telltale sign of an arrhythmia is a dramatic decline in endurance. If your regular cardio workout is suddenly a lot more exhausting, ask your doctor for an EKG. If that comes up clear, request a Holter monitor. It records your heart rhythm for 24 hours to detect more infrequent missed beats. Passing out may also be a sign of serious heart-rhythm trouble.

HOW TO DEFEND YOURSELF: One of the most common causes of arrhythmia is high blood pressure, so keep yours under 120/80 millimeters of mercury. A massage may provide pleasurable stress relief. In a recent University of South Florida study, people who underwent three 10-minute massages a week experienced an 18-point drop in their systolic blood pressure and a 5-point drop in their diastolic blood pressure after just 10 sessions.

NUMBER OF MEN HAVING A HEART ATTACK WHO DRIVE THEMSELVES TO THE HOSPITAL, WHICH IS DANGEROUS TO THEMSELVES AND THE POOR SOULS THEY RUN OVER:

1 in 14

MEDICINE'S FRONT LINE

EVERY DAY, THESE DOCTORS FIGHT FOR THE LIVES OF
AMERICAN SOLDIERS. LEARN HOW THEIR PIONEERING
TECHNIQUES MAY EVENTUALLY SAVE YOUR LIFE, TOO

BY BOB DRURY

The call comes in at 1330 hours one recent hot, dusty afternoon in the
heart of the Sunni Triangle. Ambush. A Humvee, call sign Hardrock
Six, 3rd Infantry Division, hit flush by a rocket-propelled grenade. Two
soldiers are down, one "urgent," one "priority." Urgent means loss of life,
limb, or eyesight; priority means loss of blood. Precisely 5 minutes later,
our UH-60 Black Hawk medevac lifts off from Balad Air Base, 12 miles
away. It soars over the blue-tiled roof of the mosque personally designed
by Saddam Hussein, banks left, and within seconds clears the concer-
tina wire surrounding Logistical Support Area Anaconda.

"No matter how many times you do it, you still pucker once you get
over the wire," says one of the helicopter's pilots, Chief Warrant Officer
Lance Duensing. Duensing is handsome, square-jawed, towheaded—not
quite a buzz cut. He looks as if he'd prefer to be flushing quail near his
home in the East Texas hill country. The pilot in command, Chief Warrant Officer Jackson Wood, his sunburned face as taut as a clenched
fist, throttles the aircraft, the rotors drown out conversation, and we
hurtle at 145 miles per hour toward the evacuation, or dust-off, site.

Near the Tigris River, the dull, silvery brown talc of the Iraqi desert
turns greener, wetter, burgeoning into lush fields of corn and melon
linked by irrigation ditches. Rows of date palms sprout in symmetrical
patterns on both sides of the emerald waterway, each tree capable of
concealing a man with a Kalashnikov assault rifle or a shoulder-
mounted rocket launcher. All eyes are outward except those of Specialist Elizabeth Shrode, the flight medic, who's busy arranging the blood
supply and bandages. She rechecks the oxygen tanks. Beside her, crew

chief Brandon King fingers his M-16 and scans the terrain below, his toe tapping nervously on the armor-plated floor.

From the rear seat, I steal another glance at the medic. Her brown hair is pulled back in a tight bun, and beneath her flight helmet, her dark eyeliner flatters an oval face with sharp, high cheekbones. Rifling through her first-aid kit, she appears the picture of serenity. I turn back toward the window. I pretend to be searching for snipers. It's an act. I am scared.

This is a story about a pipeline. It begins with a bullet, a chunk of shrapnel, a percussive blast attempting to suck the life out of an American soldier somewhere in Mesopotamia, and culminates on a forested hilltop in Landstuhl, Germany. It is a story about the men and women who make this remarkable medical pipeline flow—the pilots, medics, surgeons, mechanics, nurses, and litter bearers who reclaim the lives of young American soldiers who, if not for their care, would die on a battlefield far from home.

War may be the best teacher of war, as Clausewitz observed, but, from Gettysburg to Khe Sanh to Samarra, it has also been an unparalleled teacher of medicine. The rescuers in this story are aided by great leaps in modern technology, the conflict in Iraq having been the proving ground for a number of medical innovations: robotic prostheses for amputees, pills that read soldiers' vital signs, computer chips that pinpoint wounds, vacuum-sealed sterile pressure bandages, operating-room laser technology, and even a new form of antibacterial gauze with a veneer of Vaseline. All are very likely to be put to use in civilian emergency rooms across America someday.

But the primary components of this pipeline are the wisdom and heart, the dignity and valor, the expertise and dedication, of its practitioners. In many ways, this is a horrific story, as all narratives of violence visited upon youth need be. War, for all its lies, is about the truth, and no matter your view regarding the necessity or prudence of the invasion of Iraq, the fact remains that in a distant desert land, our country's soldiers are being torn to pieces at conveyer-belt rates. They would not make it home alive without this pipeline, which starts in the "golden hour," that first 60 minutes after a soldier is wounded in action, when life and death literally hang in the balance.

It starts with the medics in Balad.

In military circles, the phrase "tip of the spear" is much overused, yet it describes perfectly the medics who have rescued most of—as of this writing—the more than 16,000 U.S. servicemen and women wounded in Iraq. During the Vietnam War, it took weeks to move a wounded man from the bush to a hospital in the United States. Today, a soldier seriously wounded in Fallujah can be whisked to the Iraqi theater hospital, transferred to the American-staffed Landstuhl Medical Center in southwestern Germany, and taken to National Naval Medical Center in Bethesda, Maryland, or Walter Reed Army Medical Center in Washington, D.C., within 36 hours.

The medics at the mouth of this pipeline hail from the 54th Medical Company, out of Fort Lewis, Washington, and they're stationed at Balad Air Base, 42 miles northwest of Baghdad. This is the nexus of America's medical presence in Iraq. Located in the parched province of Salah ad Din, it's a former Iraqi Air Force base. It was captured by U.S. forces in 2003 and—with its two parallel, 11,000-foot runways—has become America's air hub in the region. The site is dusty and gritty and rocky and hot. Only a few scraggly eucalyptus trees, their leaves caked brown with sand, disrupt the endless horizon.

The base, dubbed Mortaritaville, is attached to LSA Anaconda, the U.S. Army's largest support base in Iraq. The combined, enclosed outpost, spread over an area with a 12-mile circumference, is fortified against bombardment by hundreds of asymmetrical rows of concrete blast walls, 12 to 20 feet high and 2 feet thick. They snake through the camp abutted by huge, mantrap-sized, cardboard-lined metal baskets filled with dirt, called Hesco Barriers. Roughly 20,000 soldiers and 2,800 airmen, as well as a smattering of civilian contractors and Department of Defense operators, are garrisoned there. (Members of the U.S. Air Force, man or woman, pilot or mechanic, are officially known as airmen.) They bunk in thin-skinned metal "hootches," similar to the containers that transport merchandise on ships. Each is large enough for two bed frames and two aluminum wardrobes; a few are double stacked. Though surrounded by sandbags piled 5 feet high, they offer little safety from a direct hit by a rocket or mortar, which are lobbed over the wire nightly. "Raining iron," the soldiers call it, and smile.

The neighboring Iraqi town of Balad is the heart of the remaining Saddam loyalists in Iraq. Thus, the base has a Fort Apache feel to it. Its ready-alert status requires every soldier and airman to carry or wear the bulky 4-pound Kevlar helmet and 35-pound armor-plated vest ("battle rattle") at all times, be it to the chow hall, the makeshift gym, the basketball courts, or the latrine in the middle of the night.

The 54th Medical Company's flight crews are constantly in the air, averaging 25 dust-offs and medical-supply runs a day. They take pride in the fact that they are the only medevac choppers in theater to fly without escorts. A half dozen of the 54th's Black Hawks are stationed at Balad—another half dozen are spread about the theater at smaller forward operating bases—and can cover a 50-mile radius ("60 to 70 in a pinch," says one pilot). They do not lack for business.

The aircraft, configured to carry up to six litters, have been modified into flying emergency rooms, set up for any medical contingency one might encounter in a bloody war. Their holds are crammed with oxygen tanks, blood packs, heart-rate monitors, chest and intubation tubes, pressure infusers, splints, defibrillation paddles, drugs of every stripe. It is not unusual for medics to pick up a wounded soldier at the point of impact and begin measuring his heart rate with a portable electrocardiogram machine or sedating him with a Valium infusion as the helicopter races to the field hospital.

But the bulk of a medic's work is done on the ground. It is too often sad and bloody and dangerous, all at the same time. One morning, soon after my arrival in theater, a medevac call came in after another Humvee attack in a nearby village, this vehicle blown onto its side by an IED, military shorthand for the ubiquitous improvised explosive devices that, along with suicide car bombs, have become the weapon of choice for the Iraqi insurgency. Two GIs were seriously wounded—one thrown clear by the blast and unconscious, the other, a turret gunner, pinned beneath the vehicle, his legs crushed.

The medics from the 54th arrived within minutes, only to discover another, unexploded IED—"about the size of a case of longneck beers"—planted 4 feet from the still-smoking Humvee. The scene was so fraught that ground troops setting up a perimeter around the wounded men did not dare venture closer than 50 yards for fear of being blown to hell themselves. The medics charged in, literally stepping back and forth over the live bomb as they worked. One tended the unconscious man, pounding his chest and administering mouth-to-mouth resuscitation, while the other attempted to extricate the gunner. Their efforts were for naught; both soldiers died at the scene.

Afterward, back at the air ambulance company's headquarters, the mood was somber. I watched as the medics blamed themselves for taking too much time to remove the turret gunner, and for failing to summon a backup medevac to pick up the unconscious soldier while they worked. One medic wept in fitful, silent heaves, surrounded by his buddies. The other went off to sit alone in the sand and pound his forehead.

Captain Michael Myers, another Black Hawk pilot, sidled up to me. We stared silently at the disconsolate medic sitting apart from everyone. "We all need time alone sometimes," he said, softly.

1337 hours, and Wood maneuvers the Black Hawk at treetop level, darting, zigzagging, pursuing a course over as many open fields as possible, the better to spot and evade snipers. A downed American helicopter, even one with a red cross adorning its bulbous nose, is a major coup for the Iraqi insurgency. Below, children race from whitewashed farms to peer up at the noisy bird, perhaps expecting to receive one of the soccer balls the medevac crews often drop as gifts. Two boys fishing from a shallow punt in the slow-moving Tigris give a desultory wave. To the northeast, perhaps a mile distant, two small, single-engine Kiowa Warrior helicopters armed with laser Hellfire missiles flit like dragonflies about a whitish gray plume of smoke. This is the point of impact. The flight crew does not know if the landing zone is still hot. No matter. They will try to set our aircraft down for no longer than 10 minutes. "Load and go" is the objective.

"We're in and out, no buts," the medic Sergeant Gerry Bickett had warned me earlier as we clambered into his helicopter. Bickett, tall, broad, hard as a sandbag, is nicknamed the Angry Medic. He drove home his point by jabbing a thick finger into my chest. "You fly with us and wander off, and we got the wounded loaded but we don't got you? Sayonara, we leave without you. You get some car speeding up and throwing a grenade into the bird. Or somebody in the bushes with an RPG (rocket-propelled grenade). Don't need that. Understood?" I nodded.

Bickett told me that the 54th had flown more than 3,000 medevac missions during this, its second tour in Iraq. (The 54th's 11-month tour ended late last November, a few weeks after my visit.) He could count on his fingers, he said, the number of times they'd put down longer than 10 minutes. One of those occasions, said fellow medic Tomas Chavez, had occurred at the scene of a Humvee ambush-turned-firefight outside the northern city of Kirkuk. Chavez reluctantly recounted the story as Bickett swore under his breath at the memory.

Chavez's crew had arrived to find the driver of the Humvee dead, "his head barely attached by little bits of muscle." Another soldier was wounded, critical but treatable, after having been run over by a second American vehicle in the confusion of the gunfight. A bullet had severed the femoral artery of a third soldier, Chavez's priority. "He looked about 14," the medic said. "I'm kneeling in this spreading pool of his blood, reaching up into his gut looking for the artery, trying to see if I could feel any bleeding against my fingers in there, and this kid, ghost-white pale, he keeps grabbing my hand and repeating, 'Don't let me die. Don't let me die.'

"I'm pushing his hand away, reaching in, trying to put some pressure on the severed artery. But I knew when you lose that much blood . . ." Chavez's voice trailed off. Bickett walked away, head down, muttering.

"That was one day we were on the ground for more than 10 minutes," Chavez said finally. "The boy died. It sucks. I had nightmares for months. Remembering this kid holding my hand. 'Don't let me die.' Jesus." Chavez shook his head violently, like a wet dog. "That's the exception, though."

I'm reminded of his words as, at 1339, exactly 4 minutes after liftoff, we close in on the cloud of smoke from the blasted Humvee. The Kiowa helicopters loom larger. Below, I catch sight of Abrams tanks and Bradley fighting vehicles tearing down one-lane dirt paths, throwing up gouts of dust as they race toward the point of impact. Two more soldiers down.

U.S. Air Force Balad theater hospital, one typical night: Helicopter rotors slice the desert air, the sound reverberating like the clang of a sword. The aircraft hover in tiered formation, waiting, in turn, to land. A constant procession of two-wheeled, metal rickshawlike litters streams into the emergency room. The ambulatory are herded into a corner area, while doctors, nurses, and medical technicians toting chest tubes, wound kits, bandages, anesthesia, antibiotics, and emergency airway tubes swarm the litter-bound, five or six to a patient. They break into teams, depending on wounds. Orthopedic surgeons with vascular specialists; neurosurgeons with ophthalmologists; heart surgeons with facial-recon-struction experts. The most desperate patients are stabilized, priori-tized—for the trauma ward, for ICU, for surgery. In heartbreaking situations, some are marked "expectant," as in, expected to die.

From Tikrit, a specialist E-4 is wheeled in, a member of the New Hampshire National Guard, his head swollen grotesquely from a gun-shot wound. Next, from Balad city, a GI who has taken a rocket-propelled grenade to the chest and looks as though he has passed through a wood chipper. Two Marines follow, from Anbar province, vic-tims of an IED blast. Blood drips from too many wounds to count. "How's my buddy?" croaks the one still conscious. After him, another army grunt, looking no older than 15, his left arm gone, his torso and legs punctured by shrapnel. Followed by a burly soldier, another spe-cialist E-4, his right leg hanging by sinews, his left arm swathed in bandages that reek of rotted flesh. It reminds me of a charnel house, men torn to pieces.

An Australian army chief of nurses stands at the tent entrance, track-ing the patient and resource flow. Behind him, unscathed soldiers emerge from the night, shuffling their feet, worried, sad, pissed off, their rifles on safety. They have come to check on squad mates, to volunteer to give blood. Med techs race out of the E.R. with dirty instruments, rush back in with sanitized ones. Litter bearers bend to scoop up soiled desert camouflage uniforms, bandages cut from torn bodies. More stop to sop up puddles of blood. The smell of putrid, dying muscle and tissue is almost visible. It mixes with the rubbery odor of fluids used to clean wounds, to fill intravenous tubes. No one shouts or hollers. Still, authoritative voices, sharp enough to cut falling silk, pierce the din.

"Need x-rays right here, now!"

"Just frags, soft-tissue damage. Wheel him aside."

"Out of the way, move, move, move; body coming through."

"Internal blood pooling. Sonar scan, please."

Air Force Colonel Elisha Powell IV, MD, the hospital's commanding officer, locks eyes with me. "Drury! *Men's Health*! Over here. Little help." Given the frenzy, I find his catch-in-the-throat baritone incongruously calm. "Talk to this soldier."

It is the burly GI close to losing his leg. His face is peppered with shrapnel, his front teeth missing, his lips swollen. I read his name off his chart, stroke his unbandaged right hand. "Charles, Charles, it'll be okay. You're going to be all right. Charles? You hear me, Charles?"

"Hell'm I doin' here?" he rasps. He is from the California National Guard. Blown out of the turret of his Humvee by an IED while conducting a raid in south Baghdad.

"Charles, listen to me. These docs are the best, man. The best. Fix you up like new."

Dr. Powell, an orthopedic surgeon, bends over the soldier's shattered leg and says, without looking up, "Gonna get you on the cover of *Men's Health*, Charles."

I say, "That's right, Charles, get you on the cover."

With this, the slits of Charles's hot red eyes open almost imperceptibly. He turns his head. "No way, man. Ain't got the abs." Then the IV of Valium tenders oblivion.

"O.R. 3 is open," someone says.

"I need it!"

Like this, for hours.

The Balad theater hospital, the busiest frontline medical facility since the Vietnam War, resembles nothing so much as a Bactrian bazaar. Two rows of parallel, 64- x 20-foot interconnected tents extending 300 yards have been laid over a concrete slab in the shape of a giant letter H. The double-corridored canvas structure, connected by a middle passageway, houses a large emergency room, a pharmacy lab (with a mobile isolation chamber capable of mixing drugs such as antibiotics or insulin drips in a sterile environment), multiple recovery wards (for Americans, allied combatants, Iraqi civilians, and enemy wounded), warrens of offices, storage rooms, and nonmedical tents used as a conference room, small chow hall, and admitting office. Its six operating rooms are its only hardened facilities, built to withstand a mortar attack.

One night, a wounded GI, his arm in a sling, stubs out his smoke and asks me if I know the name of the doctor in pale blue scrubs standing outside the door to the tented emergency room. "I swear that's the guy who brought me in," he says. It is, in fact, Tomas Chavez, who, when not flying dust-offs, volunteers as a physician's assistant in the hospital's emergency and operating rooms. After Chavez and the wounded soldier exchange greetings, I sit down with the medic, who is emblematic of the symbiotic nature of the U.S. military's medical pipeline.

With his dark, brooding features and big coal eyes, Chavez, 30, is ribbed by his fellow medics as the Erik Estrada of the 54th. He's the oldest son of Mexican immigrants who settled in Tempe, Arizona. The first in his family to attend college, he was a senior majoring in premed when the 9/11 attacks occurred. He interrupted his schooling to enlist in the army and, like his fellow medics, before being deployed to Iraq was put through courses in trauma medicine, emergency medical skills, and Special Forces medical training. He intends to enroll in the University of Arizona's medical school when his 4-year enlistment is up.

He says what he has learned assisting the doctors at the hospital has been invaluable out in the field. In the operating room, he may intubate the airway of one patient, remove small pieces of shrapnel from the flesh and bone of another. "Everything I do in there just gives me that much more confidence on a dust-off," he says. "It's the same for every medic I work with."

The operating rooms are the hospital's only sterilized shells, and as Chavez and I now walk the dusty hallways, he takes informal inventory of the new medical technology that war naturally breeds. We pass areas laden with a pharmacopoeia of drugs, rooms stacked floor to ceiling with boxes of blood, QuickClot clotting agent, "clingy" gauze, and vacuum-sealed pressure bandages. "But new doesn't always mean better," he says, demonstrating how an older, plastic-hinged tourniquet outperforms its modern metal counterpart. "And the old standbys never go away," he adds, patting his flak vest and producing several tampons from his pockets. "Can't beat them for jamming into bullet holes."

Chavez and his fellow medics fear that now that the enemy knows the American battle rattle is keeping soldiers alive by protecting their vital organs, they will raise the ante. "We're already seeing a lot more burn victims. They've learned about the armor plating, so they're packing their IEDs with detergent, oil, and gasoline," he says.

"My first tour, I figured you never know what you're gonna find at the point of impact: soldiers trapped in burning vehicles, firefights, bodies blasted by IEDs," Chavez continues. "But now, after two tours, it pretty much comes down to finding one thing: anybody who's still alive. Then making sure they're still alive by the time you get 'em back to base."

Chavez pauses. "Don't paint us the heroes," he finally says. "We only go out and get 'em. It's the air-force docs in the base hospital who keep 'em alive."

It's well past midnight. Outside, beneath a starless canopy, Dr. Powell, exhausted, satisfied, sighs. "Didn't lose one tonight," he says. This is routine. Ninety-six percent of the wounded who arrive alive at Balad theater hospital to be treated by the Air Force's 332nd Expeditionary Medical Group survive. Dr. Powell is taking a moment to introduce me and photographer Max Becherer to the Swamp, a grimy, pillboxlike structure adjacent to the hospital, where he and his surgeons catch catnaps between shifts. They have named it in homage to the living quarters of the characters Hawkeye Pierce and Trapper John on *M*A*S*H*.

"It's all about speed. That's the biggest difference in saving lives in this war," he says. "We call it the Del Rio model, after a small town in West Texas about 150 miles from our stateside base in San Antonio. When you get hurt in Del Rio, there are lots of little community hospitals between Del Rio and San Antonio. But you shouldn't stop there if you have a severe trauma. You want to go right to San Antonio. The medics know it, the pilots know it. Don't make the intermediary stop. It's a waste of time, and time is precious."

Twenty-five minutes is the average time elapsed between a point-of-impact dust-off and a wounded patient's arrival in a Balad operating room. This includes stops for emergency-room triage, portable CAT scans, digitized computer x-rays, and sonar-imaging scans that detect internal bleeding.

Although it lacks Hawkeye's still, the Swamp does have a tar-beach roof to which the medicos now retire to sit in rickety beach chairs and smoke thick, pungent cigars. The roof overlooks the perimeter wire, the pitch-black "real Iraq" not 20 feet away. Dr. Powell offers me a cigar, reads my thoughts. "Keep the glowing end cupped in your hand," he says.

My eyes drift toward the wire, with its canal berm offering natural cover. "It only takes one," says Becherer.

"Think of the mortars as lightning," shrugs Major Corey Harrison, MD, a redheaded E.R. specialist from New York. His body armor is smeared with dried blood. "If it's your turn, it's your turn. Nothing you can do."

Balad hospital is staffed by a remarkable collection of air-force surgeons and trauma-care doctors, aided by a few army or navy practitioners, as well as multinational auxiliaries (Aussie nurses, Iraqi interpreters). The medical group includes four orthopedic surgeons, two neurosurgeons, six trauma surgeons, a facial-reconstruction specialist, a heart surgeon, a urologist, a vascular surgeon, two hand surgeons, and an ophthalmologist. Their pedigrees form an impressive roster: Ivy League universities, Georgetown, Notre Dame, and (like Dr. Powell himself) the Air Force Academy.

"Even with an unlimited budget, I couldn't buy in private practice the team I have here now," says Dr. Powell. He screws up the features on his hawklike face, and a sudden breeze rustles his salt-and-pepper hair. "Not at the Mayo Clinic, not at the Hospital for Special Surgery in New York. Nowhere."

"Back in the States, we'd be at each other's throats," adds Colonel Jack Ingari, MD, a Harvard graduate, the hospital's second in command, and

one of the nation's foremost microscopic-vascular-surgery hand specialists. He laughs. "Who's making more money? Who's the top dog? Who's
the lead surgeon and who's the assistant?

"Jeez," he continues, "there'd be scalpels in people's backs."

"As corny as it sounds, over here it's a higher calling," says Dr. Powell.
"No one in an emergency room back in the States sees in 6 months what
we see here in one night. Most of the things I've seen here—the huge
blast wounds, the head injuries, the amputations, the open fractures—
I'll never see again in my professional career."

Now the conversation ceases, and several surgeons prick their ears
toward the night sky. Somewhere in the distance, the muffled beat of a
helicopter's rotors ruffle the air. The doctors stand as one, douse their
cigars. "They say medicine is a marathon," Dr. Powell says. "Well, out
here it's a sprint."

Around 5 o'clock the following evening, I witness Dr. Powell and Dr.
Ingari performing a delicate procedure on a soldier whose leg has been
shattered by an IED. It is called an internal fixation. After drilling a
hole down to the marrow in one end of the boy's femur, the doctors
insert a steel rod through the length of the broken bone and hold it
together by tightening screws through precut holes in the rod. The device
keeps the long bone from moving or shortening as it mends, and a drain
is left in the wound to collect excess blood and lower infection risk.

"This is something that's never been done in field hospitals before,"
says Dr. Powell. "Normally, a patient would have to wait until Landstuhl, or even the States, because no one would think to do it in the
field. But we've got people here innovative enough to perform all sorts
of new procedures, and I guarantee you that the one thing that will
come out of this war, besides the technological advances, will be the
experience that we're pumping through this system. These surgeons
and nurses and enlisted techs are going to be the ones who carry America's health-care system through future mass-casualty events."

He sweeps his hand in the direction of the emergency room. "The
young doctors you see out there? They'll be the leaders in their medical
communities when they get out. They'll be the folks teaching everybody

at our medical centers and our medical schools and our trauma hospitals for the next 20 years. No one else will have this experience."

To punctuate his remarks, the base's warning siren sounds, and a recorded voice intones, "Incoming. Incoming. Incoming." In the E.R., medical staffers nonchalantly lay aside scalpels, intubation tubes, anesthesia drips, to don helmets and armored vests before returning to work. Somewhere on the far side of the base, four staggered mortar explosions resound. The only surprise, one trauma doctor tells me later, is that the blasts were spread out over several seconds. "Usually, they're bangbangbang."

The next morning, an explanation. The enemy has perfected a new ploy: placing mortar tubes into buckets of water, which are then frozen and planted near the wire in the middle of the night. When the morning sun melts the water, the mortars drop, hit the bottom of the metal buckets, and fire. Because the pails vary in size, the water melts at different rates, producing the staggered firing effect.

A few hours later, two Iraqi boys are delivered to the Balad theater hospital by a medevac from the 54th. Gerry Bickett, cursing, carries one in. Ten-year-old playmates from a village near the Syrian border, they'd stumbled across a small, unexploded IED, picked it up to examine it, and thrown it away. That's when it exploded, raking them both with shrapnel and breaking the leg of one child. The boys' fathers have accompanied them on the Black Hawk, and as the two slight, nervous men pace the emergency room in their soiled dishdashas, Dr. Powell and Dr. Ingari operate immediately.

Afterward, over coffee, I ask the 44-year-old Dr. Powell, still wearing his surgical scrubs, how often he is reminded of his own children back in San Antonio. "Sometimes you feel a tremendous amount of pressure, but to be an effective surgeon, you have to compartmentalize those feelings," he says.

"I have to focus on saving these patients' lives, be they Iraqi or American kids, rather than dwell on the fact that I have a 12-year-old boy and a 10-year-old girl back home.

"Our patients don't have time for us to feel sorry for them," he goes on. "They come to us to fix them, to repair their fractures, to close their wounds, to make them better. If I start thinking that this could be my son or my daughter . . . let's just say they don't want us to feel sorry for them. They want us to patch them up and get them back to their units."

Or to Germany.

Combat takeoff, 0300. The cavernous C-17 Globemaster cargo jet taxis, picks up speed, and shoots into the coal black sky like a rocket. Through the dim, red blackout lights, I watch as the head nurse, maintaining her balance while wearing 40 pounds of Kevlar, monitors the machines attached to the six litter-bound patients strapped onto metal cots. Most are unconscious. Eleven additional soldiers, walking wounded who are armored, helmeted, and belted into fold-down chairs lining both sides of the windowless fuselage, brace themselves against gravity. The C-17's pilots will take stomach-twisting evasive action to 24,000 feet, level off at 30,000 feet, and turn on the lights once they have escaped Iraqi airspace.

If a combat landing on an Iraqi airstrip is comparable to being a passenger in a kamikaze dive-bomber, the combat takeoff, says U.S. Air Force Lieutenant Colonel Scott Van De Hoef, MD, "is like being strapped to the back of a giant arrow shot straight into the air."

A few hours earlier, Dr. Van De Hoef and I had stood alongside the Balad flight line in the shadow of the CASF's tented facility, where the physician works. CASF stands for Contingency Aeromedical Staging Facility, and, as Dr. Van De Hoef explained, "I guess you'd describe us, in baseball terms, as kind of like a middle reliever, the bridge between the starters at Balad and the closers in Landstuhl."

Dr. Van De Hoef, 36, a Florida family practitioner, has a soft smile and an easy wit, although at the moment we spoke, humor seemed antithetical to the point. He and his medical team had just finished lifting a horribly burned soldier through the yawning clamshell of a C-17, where his life-support system would be monitored by a critical-care air-transport team (CCATT) during the 5-hour flight to Ramstein Air Base in Germany. Each CCATT consists of a trauma surgeon, flight nurse, and respiratory technician.

The burned GI had been delivered from the theater hospital to the

PERCENTAGE OF MEN WHO SAY THEY FEAR DEATH:

35

air transport by a CASF ambulance bus and carried into the jet with what looked like a desktop computer resting on his chest. "Packaging the patient," it's called, and it consists of a ventilator, a cardiac monitor, a blood-oxygen monitor, vacuum suction tubes to keep wounds clean, and a blood-pressure monitor. If the Black Hawk medevac helicopters are flying emergency rooms, the CCATT flights are movable ICUs. When necessary, an Air-Evac flight can accommodate 36 litters, stacked three high on stanchions.

I asked Dr. Van De Hoef about the frequency of the Air-Evac flights out of Balad, considering that injured soldiers are typically whisked out of the hospital within 24 hours. He ran a finger down the sheaf of paper attached to the clipboard he was holding. "I've had wounded soldiers from everywhere in Iraq come through here for . . . let's see . . . Sorry, this register only goes back 8 weeks. But in that time, we've loaded over 100 flights, more than 1,300 patients. You can extrapolate a year's worth." (It works out to about 8,000 living patients a year. Battle dead are shipped home directly on separate flights.) He shook his head slowly. "You only hope you can do right by the families who can't be here when you're taking care of their kids. Last week, we had a kid come through, his face looked familiar, and I thought I recognized the name. I asked him, 'Didn't I just send you out of here?' He goes, 'No, that was my brother.' "

Tonight's Air-Evac crew, an amalgam of Mississippi National Guard airmen and German-based air-force medical staff, have their hands full during the uneventful flight to Ramstein Air Base. The nurses hustle from litter to litter, monitoring and remonitoring the myriad machines recording the vital signs of the wounded.

At Ramstein, the wounded exit the plane in a teeming rain—carried, limping, walking—and are transported from the American air base via blue ambulance buses to the circular drive outside the Landstuhl Medical Center's emergency room. Employing a "joint tracking system," medical personnel in Germany are already aware of the specific treatment each injured soldier requires, be it burn care or the management of brain injuries, bullet wounds, or amputated limbs.

An air-force chaplain outside the hospital positions himself to be the first to speak to any conscious soldiers coming off the bus. "We've been praying for you since you were injured," he says. Off to one side, I spy several American nurses near a smoking kiosk, their eyes rimmed in red. I learn that they are mourning the passing of a patient, a young soldier who was kept alive on a ventilator long enough for his parents to fly in from the United States and watch him receive his Purple Heart.

"We have empathy, but we can't have sympathy," one tells me. "We'd fall apart." Her swollen eyes belie her words.

"Compassion fatigue—it happens to all of us," says U.S. Air Force Major Tim Woods, MD, the lanky 38-year-old general surgeon whom I accompany on his rounds through the intensive-care unit at Landstuhl Medical Center. "Sometimes you start thinking about how overwhelming it all is."

The Landstuhl facility, the largest American military hospital outside the United States, sits atop a small mountain overlooking the town of the same name. Staffed jointly by about 2,000 army and air-force medical personnel, the 162-bed medical center is bounded by dark, wet hills blanketed by maple, black locust, and birch. Although a quarter of its multinational patients arrive with hard-core battle injuries from Iraq and Afghanistan—"down range," as the war zones are called—the hospital is, aesthetically, far enough from Balad to be on another planet.

That is, until you encounter its patients. In one room, Dr. Woods introduces me to the burn victim, a kid in his early 20s whose only request is to be "made whole enough" to rejoin his unit. Dr. Woods asks me not to follow him into a second room. Inside is a boy, unconscious on the bed, the victim of an RPG attack. "He's not going to make it," Dr. Woods says.

The doctor describes Landstuhl as a "stabilizing and reconnecting" facility. "In Balad, they stop the bleeding, save the patient's life," he says. "Here, we get them on the road to rehab and recovery that, hopefully, continues back in the States." (All patients who are wounded in action and sent to Landstuhl head home from here; 22 percent eventually make it back to their units.) Any patient not confined to a ventilator at Landstuhl

(continued on page 196)

A WOUNDED SOLDIER'S JOURNEY

Elapsed Time: 00:00 Point of Impact

A soldier is down, seriously wounded. More than half the time, the rescue call goes to the air-ambulance company stationed at Balad Air Base, 42 miles northwest of Baghdad and home to the most advanced hospital in the combat zone. When *Men's Health* visited in November 2005, the evacuation of injured soldiers was the responsibility of the 54th Medical Company. During a typical 24-hour period, the 54th flew 13 rescue missions with its six Black Hawk medevac helicopters, transporting an average of 20 American soldiers back to Balad hospital, along with several coalition and Iraqi troops.

00:18 Arrival at Balad Hospital

Balad hospital, run by the 332nd Expeditionary Medical Group, provides state-of-the-art care. More than half of the patients who come through the hospital have injuries so severe that they're at risk of death or disability. In previous conflicts many of these soldiers wouldn't have survived. But today's helmets and body armor—layers of Kevlar fortified with ceramic plates—are impervious to bullets and shrapnel, keeping vital organs safe. Soldiers who make it as far as Balad have a 96 percent survival rate, though amputations are double those of the previous Gulf War. In fact, almost 88 percent of soldiers evacuating Balad have injuries to the arms or legs.

00:25 Emergency Room and Triage

The first stop for a wounded soldier is the E.R. The most desperately injured are stabilized and moved to an operating room or the trauma intensive-care unit. Others are prioritized by the seriousness of their injuries and sent to the trauma ICU or a 40-bed intermediate-care facility.

00:35 Surgery

The 50 doctors of the 332nd Expeditionary Medical Group specialize in two dozen types of medicine, from neurosurgery to infectious disease. They perform an average of 26 surgical procedures a day—half are "major," with a soldier's life on the line. Forty percent are done on U.S. military personnel, the rest on Iraqi soldiers and civilians. This is because American soldiers are usually sent to Germany for follow-up surgery; Iraqi troops stay at Balad until they're well enough to go home.

02:30 Recovery

After surgery, wounded soldiers recuperate in the 18-bed intensive-care unit and recovery room. American and coalition troops who will be well enough to return to their units within 2 weeks stay in Balad to recover. Those who won't be able to return to active duty—or who'll need longer than 2 weeks to recover—are airlifted to Landstuhl Medical Center, in Germany, as soon as they're stable enough to fly.

In preparation for the 5-hour flight to Germany, medics "pack" the litters of the most seriously wounded with ventilators and various monitors, then transport them by bus to a waiting C-17 cargo plane.

12:00 Evacuation to Landstuhl, Germany

The 332nd Expeditionary Medical Group runs the busiest Contingency Aeromedical Staging Facility (CASF) in the world. Not only are Balad patients evacuated from here, but so are soldiers from the dozen other hospitals across Iraq. The C-17 Globemaster cargo jet can hold as many as 36 litter patients, though the average is 24. About two evacuees per flight are classified as critical-care patients—that is, to survive, they need medical care on the plane.

18:00 Arrival at Landstuhl

It's a 5-hour flight to Ramstein Air Base in Germany, where the injured soldiers are transferred by ambulance bus to Landstuhl Medical Center, 8 miles away.

19:00 Evaluation

With 162 beds, Landstuhl is the largest American-run hospital outside the United States. (By comparison, Massachusetts General Hospital has 893 beds.) About 30 injured soldiers arrive here daily—not only battle wounded from Iraq and Afghanistan, but also sick or wounded servicemen from Europe or Asia.

31:00 Discharge to the States

Three military flights a week connect Ramstein Air Base and Andrews Air Force Base in Maryland, and an average of 23 wounded soldiers arrive home on these flights each week. (Dead soldiers travel separately on direct flights that originate in Iraq and land at Dover Air Force Base in Delaware.)

36:00 Arrival

After arriving at Andrews, soldiers are transferred to Walter Reed Medical Center in Washington, D.C., or the National Naval Medical Center in Bethesda, Maryland. As bad as their physical injuries are, the mental scars can be worse. Three out of 10 Iraq veterans show signs of mental stress within 4 months, and 17 percent are diagnosed with post-traumatic stress disorder. What's more, one in five married soldiers faces divorce within 2 years of being deployed, and 15 percent of vets develop depression.

begins physical rehab immediately upon arrival. It's not as easy as it sounds. There are amputees' bones to be beveled and skin grafts to be performed. Immune systems are weak, and viral pneumonias and bacterial infections rage.

But at the end of the day, Dr. Woods says, it's the speed with which the wounded arrive in his ward that holds him most in thrall. "That's the most important and amazing medical advance of this war."

I cannot share his enthusiasm, I admit to him. I have seen more than enough of the torn and shattered young victims who constitute this pipeline. He nods. "I know. I see these kids coming in, half my age, just blown to hell. Rips up my insides."

Dust-off site, 1340. The Black Hawk medevac puts down in a blinding cloud of dirt and grit. It has taken us exactly 5 minutes to get here, an arid soccer field abutting a small cluster of flat brown houses. Medic Elizabeth Shrode and crew chief Brandon King heave two litters from the helicopter's side door. Shrode dashes toward an inert body, splayed perhaps 20 yards from the idling helicopter. King, tethered by a radio cord, stops several feet from the Black Hawk, drops to one knee, swivels his M-16 in an arcing motion.

Ground troops from a nearby Bradley fighting vehicle rush to meet Shrode, now bent over the fallen soldier. He has short, blond curls. He does not look much older than my 8-year-old son. His face, a death mask, has gone gray. Shrode feels his wrist, searching for a pulse. She drops his arm and places her fingers against his neck. Blood pools in the sand. He is lifted onto a litter. Most of his insides spill onto the ground. Only now do I realize that his feet are facing backward. He has been blown in half, his body held together only by his belt and uniform pants.

Shrode turns, yells something to the ground troops. She is looking for the second soldier. There were supposed to be two: one urgent; one priority. The platoon leader on the ground appears confused. He races back to the Bradley, picks up a field telephone. Using hand signals, he indicates that the dead boy on the litter is alone. Shrode and three GIs lift the body onto the Black Hawk. King covers them. We lift off again at

1345. Just 5 minutes on the ground. We arrive at the Balad theater hospital 5 minutes later. There is no urgency to the flight.

Back at the 54th's headquarters, a maintenance team immediately begins the task of power-washing blood from the aircraft. The crew huddles in a semicircle. No one says a word. I walk away. Sergeant Joe Renteria, the company's medical-standardization instructor and, at 31, the wise man of the outfit, approaches me.

"You okay?" he asks.

"Oughta see to your crew," I say.

"I'm seeing to you."

"Kid didn't look much older than my son."

"You can't take it personally."

I look up at him.

"We got the best track record in the army," he goes on. "We bring 'em back alive . . . almost all the time."

INDULGE YOUR SWEET TOOTH

While you're probably aware that it's heart healthy, chocolate may be even more powerful than previously thought, a new study reports. When Dutch scientists followed nearly 500 men for 15 years, they found that those who ate the most cocoa daily had a 50 percent lower risk of dying of heart disease than those who ate the least.

"Antioxidants in cocoa activate nitric oxide, an enzyme that relaxes blood vessels, making it easier for your heart to deliver blood throughout your body," says lead researcher Brian Buijsse, MSc. The most surprising finding? The death-defying benefits were achieved by consuming just 4 grams of cocoa a day—about the same amount as in two chocolate Hershey's Kisses.

TRY MULTITASKING MEDICINE

Choose the right blood-pressure drug and it may help thwart heart disease and diabetes, too, according to a new study in the *Lancet*. As part of a 5-year investigation, researchers treated more than 19,000 hypertensive patients with either a calcium channel blocker or a beta-blocker. Over time, people taking the calcium channel blocker were 30 percent less likely to develop diabetes, 16 percent less likely to have a heart attack, and 23 percent less likely to suffer a stroke, compared with those on beta-blockers. If you have high blood pressure and a family history of heart disease or diabetes, ask your MD about this multipurpose medication.

CHECK YOUR MIRROR FOR DIABETES RISK

Look at your eyebrows. Those two caterpillars on your forehead could save your life. Eyebrow color may reveal your risk of diabetes, say German researchers, who came to their conclusion after examining the blood-sugar levels of 100 men with gray hair. Of the men with dark eyebrows, 76 percent had diabetes, compared with just 18 percent of the gray-browed group.

"Diabetes may cause a delay or inhibition of graying in the eyebrow hair follicles," says Uwe Wollina, MD, PhD, the lead study author. If your hair is turning gray but your eyebrows are still dark, ask your doctor for a fasting glucose test: Levels above 100 milligrams per deciliter indicate a high risk of diabetes.

Also check your inseam. Having short legs could indicate a higher risk of type-2 diabetes, say Johns Hopkins University researchers. After measuring the bodies and glucose levels of 3,600 men, they discovered that those with legs shorter than 32 inches were 34 percent more likely to develop diabetes than longer-limbed men. The link may stem from poor childhood nutrition or irregular levels of a hormone called insulin-like growth factor-I. If your inseams are less than 32 inches, get a fasting glucose test.

FIGHT DISEASE WITH FLAX

When researchers at Harvard University compared the diets of 38,378 men with their rates of disease over 10 years, the scientists discovered that a 1-gram increase in daily intake of alpha-linolenic acid (ALA) can reduce a man's risk of developing pneumonia by 31 percent.

ALA is an omega-3 fat that helps decrease infection risk by quelling inflammation and regulating blood sugar, says study author Anwar Merchant, PhD. Get your extra gram by eating vegetables or chicken sautéed in a tablespoon of canola oil, or by mixing 2 teaspoons of ground flaxseed into your protein shake. (You can find flaxseed in the health-food section of your grocery store.)

HARNESS THE POWER OF PROTEIN

Even small dietary tweaks can help your heart, reports a new study published in the *Journal of the American Medical Association*. When people on low-fat diets replaced just 10 percent of their carbohydrate intake with protein, they decreased their blood pressure, triglycerides, and LDL (bad) cholesterol—reducing heart-disease risk by 13 percent. That's the equivalent of trading 60 grams of carbohydrates—the amount in one bagel—for two servings of turkey, chicken, fish, or beef. (One serving of meat is about the size of a deck of cards.)

SAVE YOURSELF WITH SANKA

If part of the way you misspent your youth was by smoking, start drinking decaffeinated coffee now. In a study of 993 former smokers, researchers at Roswell Park Cancer Institute in Buffalo, New York, found that those who consumed at least 2 cups of decaf daily were 36 percent less likely to develop lung cancer than those who drank caffeinated black tea or coffee.

Researchers aren't sure why drinking decaf helps limit the cancerous consequences of smoking but credit coffee beans' high levels of flavonoids, which prevent the DNA damage that can cause tumors to take hold. "Caffeine has been shown to reduce flavonoids' beneficial effects," notes lead researcher Kirsten Moysich, PhD.

PERCENTAGE MORE LIKELY YOU ARE TO SUFFER A STROKE OR HEART ATTACK ON YOUR BIRTHDAY THAN ANY OTHER DAY: 27

STRIVE FOR FIVE

People who eat more than five servings of fruits and vegetables a day have a 26 percent lower risk of stroke than those who eat less than three servings, according to a new U.K. study. A simple way to boost your intake? Eat a piece of fresh fruit—like an apple—on your way to work every day.

DRINK MORE BEER

Another reason to love beer: Researchers in Italy recently determined that xanthohumol, an antioxidant found in abundance in hops, can inhibit the growth of cancer cells, slowing tumor development. So far, the results have been shown only in test tubes, but human studies are planned.

ROOT OUT A KILLER

Sometimes a farmer can do what big pharma can't. Case in point: Produce helps prevent pancreatic cancer, according to new research from the University of California at San Francisco. When scientists tracked the diets of more than 2,000 people over a 10-year period, they found that eating a diet rich in fruits and vegetables cuts the chance of developing this especially deadly form of cancer by 50 percent.

"The foods most strongly associated with risk reduction are onions and garlic, beans, carrots, dark leafy vegetables, cruciferous vegetables, and oranges," says study author Elizabeth A. Holly, PhD, MPH. So eat up: People who ate five servings of vegetables a day had the lowest risk.

DROP YOUR DEAD WEIGHT

You can now add cancer to the long list of reasons to slim down. When U.K. researchers tracked 17,000 men for nearly 30 years, they found that increases in body-mass index were directly proportional to the likelihood of dying of cancers of the gut—specifically, rectal, bladder, colon, or liver cancer. Eating too many calories may lead to an increase in insulin-like growth factor (IGF-I), a hormone that encourages tumor growth, notes study author David Batty, PhD. Taking in less sugar and processed carbohydrates such as white bread, white rice, and pasta is the best way to control IGF-I levels—as well as spark weight loss.

A MORE PRECISE PROSTATE TEST

The debate over PSA testing may soon be moot, thanks to a new detection tool being designed at the University of Michigan. The blood test measures levels of 22 biomarkers that point to the presence of prostate cancer. In lab studies, the test was 93 percent accurate, compared with 80 percent for the PSA test. Clinical trials are planned.

BELLY FAT STEM CELLS

Blubber isn't all bad. Researchers at the University of Virginia have discovered that the abdominal fat collected from liposuction procedures may be a good source of stem cells. It seems fat cells may be uniquely suited to growing blood vessels, heart muscle, nerves, and bone marrow.

HIGH-SPEED HEAD EXAM

Minutes can mean the difference between recovering from a stroke and being brain damaged by one. That's why a British scientist is developing a portable brain scanner to help EMTs diagnose suspected stroke

NUMBER OF YEARS OF THE NEW AVERAGE LIFE EXPECTANCY FOR AMERICAN MEN:
78.1

victims in the ambulance. The helmetlike device uses Bluetooth technology to transmit an image of the brain to an onboard computer. This way, doctors can administer clot-busting drugs as soon as a patient arrives at the hospital.

SOUPED-UP BROCCOLI

If vegetables don't already qualify as superfoods, they soon will. U.K. researchers are working to breed a strain of broccoli that will contain three times more sulforaphane, a chemical found in cruciferous vegetables that's been linked to cancer prevention in numerous test-tube studies. The researchers hope to have the new broccoli on the market within a few years.

SKIN TEST FOR ALZHEIMER'S DISEASE

You don't need your head examined to diagnose your risk of Alzheimer's disease—a skin sample will do. NIH researchers measured levels of a protein called Erk in 60 skin-cell samples and found them to be more accurate at detecting Alzheimer's than current techniques. Researchers are trying to make the test available in doctors' offices.

LIVE LONGER

FIVE DEATH-DEFYING STRATEGIES

1. **SWALLOW A BITTER PILL:** Harvard research shows that people who ate chocolate just once a month lived longer than abstainers, probably because of the antioxidants in dark chocolate. When you choose a dark bar, look for the percentage of cacao; the higher the number, the more antioxidants hiding inside. (Bitterness also increases with cacao content, so go with the max your taste buds can bear.) **+ 1 year**

2. **GET IN THE GAME:** Japanese researchers found that men who were still involved in sports at age 65 outlived their inactive counter-parts. Credit the combination of exercise and social interaction. Join an organized team sport—like softball or basketball, not bowling—and the peer pressure to play may keep you from rotting in a rocking chair. **+2 years**

3. **STOP YOUR WORRYING:** You'll enjoy life more and have more life to enjoy: A recent study of more than 6,000 Chicago residents by the Rush Institute for Healthy Aging determined that those who were the least anxious on a day-to-day basis lived the longest. Why? A constant state of stress has been shown to undermine the immune system. Distract your one-track mind with a brain game like Sudoku. **+2 years**

4. **SHOW UP ON SUNDAY:** Or Friday night if you're Jewish. Whenever and wherever you might worship, just do it. University of Pittsburgh

PERCENTAGE OF MEN WHO HAVE HAD A MEDICAL CHECKUP WITHIN THE PAST YEAR:

70

researchers found that weekly attendance at religious services may add years to a person's expiration date, an increase equal to that seen with statin use. Not religious? Commit to a weekly group activity that feels like a spiritual experience—like watching football. **+3 years**

5. TALK YOURSELF INTO IT: Believing you're in control of your health can be a self-fulfilling prophecy. According to a Canadian study of healthy elderly people, study participants who predicted that they would live 8 more years actually did, while those who foresaw an early funeral got exactly that. Beliefs beget actions, negative and positive. **+8 years**

I'm 46, and I had a heart attack last summer. My doctor told me to avoid rigorous sex. Am I relegated to a life of girl-on-top?

Absolutely not, although there are certainly worse fates. "Most patients can have any type of sex they want after a heart attack," says John Elefteriades, MD, chief of cardiothoracic surgery at Yale–New Haven Hospital. The disclaimer, of course, is that you check with your doctor to gauge exactly how much vigor your heart can handle. But the statistics are on your side. A study of 1,663 men by Harvard University found that the odds of someone with coronary disease having a heart attack during sex were 1 in 50,000. Another study of 918 men by the University of Bristol in England found that sex can actually reduce the risk of a heart attack; the participants who had "high orgasmic frequency" through nonvigorous sex (the kind that doesn't cause sweating or loss of breath) halved their risk of a coronary event.

To be clear, no one is recommending that you start swinging from the chandeliers. But the bottom line is that "sex is exercise, and exercise is good for the heart," says Dr. Elefteriades. If you experience chest pain or shortness of breath, though, cool your engines immediately.

Should I get a high-tech "snapshot" of my heart?

Only if you're at risk for heart disease. The "snapshot" you're referring to is probably the 64-slice CT scan, which takes pictures at a rate of 150 a second—fast enough to freeze the heart midbeat and render it in 3-D. In just 10 to 20 minutes, these scanners make data available noninvasively that would normally require a catheterization (in which a small tube is snaked from a femoral artery in one leg to a coronary artery near the heart). "It allows us to see all of the heart, inside coronary arteries, and even a portion of the lungs," says Ella Kazerooni, MD, director of the Cardiothoracic Radiology Division at the University of Michigan.

Before getting scanned, though, consider the drawbacks. First, doctors are still figuring out how to use it to diagnose and guide treatment, and if a blockage is found, you'll still need a catheterization to confirm it. Second, many insurance companies won't cover it for preventive screening, and the out-of-pocket cost for patients ranges from $750 to $2,000. Third, the scan subjects you to a high dose of radiation—equal to receiving several chest x-rays at once. Bottom line: "If you're healthy and at low risk for heart disease, there's no reason to get scanned," says Dr. Kazerooni.

Can I get heart-healthy-fat benefits from low-fat peanut butter?

Stick with regular peanut butter if you're looking to shrink your chances of heart disease. Reduced-fat varieties have about a third less of the LDL- cholesterol-lowering fat per serving, says Jo Ann Carson, PhD, a professor of clinical nutrition at the University of Texas Southwestern Medical Center. Upgrade to natural brands that are made of just peanuts and salt. These have the highest levels of monounsaturated fat, especially brands in which the pure peanut oil settles near the top of the jar. Stir in the liquid when you open the jar, then store it in the fridge. It'll stay mixed.

Zocor is going off patent. Should I switch to it?

The numbers will tell you. If you have an LDL level between 150 and 200, making the switch to simvastatin (the generic version of the statin Zocor) could save you $10 or more on your co-pay, and your results will be the same as if you were taking a more potent drug like Lipitor. "Both Zocor and Lipitor have produced tremendous improvements in risk of heart attack, stroke, and death," says Jaimie Gerber, MD, a statin researcher and assistant clinical professor of internal medicine at the Yale University School of Medicine.

But beware: If you have a family history of high cholesterol or an

LDL level over 200, making the switch could be dangerous. You'd need at least four times the amount of Zocor to equal a dose of Lipitor, and "switching cholesterol medications when your current pill is doing the job may not be appropriate," warns Dr. Gerber. Consult your doctor about how much cholesterol lowering you need and what kinds of side effects you can expect from a new medication.

My cholesterol is high. Should I try lifestyle changes or a prescription?

Maybe both, says Dr. Elefteriades. A superstrict diet will decrease it a bit, but statins will lower it more and allow some wiggle room at meals. Statins also appear to be beneficial in preventing Alzheimer's disease and aortic aneurysms.

There's a big gap between my blood pressure numbers. Is that a problem?

Yes, says Dr. Elefteriades. In adults, systolic pressure (the top number; the pressure in your blood vessels when the heart beats) should be 120 millimeters of mercury (mmHG) or less. Diastolic pressure (the bottom number; the pressure when your heart is at rest) should be 80 mmHG or less. Both numbers are important in your blood-pressure reading, and so is the difference between them.

"The two numbers should never be more than 60 points apart," Dr. Elefteriades says. "Being 70 points apart suggests there could be a deeper problem, such as a leaky valve"—a condition in which bloodflow through the heart becomes more turbulent than normal. A leaky heart valve can cause shortness of breath, weakening of the heart, and, ultimately, heart failure. Go to your doctor, and he or she will probably schedule an echocardiogram to see if you have a leaky valve.

Is it true that we all have cancer cells in our bodies right now?

No. "Everyone has cells that have mutant proteins from DNA damage, but to say that that's cancer would be alarmist," says Jennifer Loros, PhD, a professor of biochemistry and genetics at

Dartmouth Medical School. A cell's natural cycle has checkpoints when it determines whether it's in a healthy state and should divide, or is damaged and should repair or kill itself.

"Cancer can occur when the normal checkpoints in the cell cycle are misregulated somehow and the [unhealthy] cell starts dividing," Loros says. Usually, a powerful protein called P-53 will trigger tumor suppression if damage is detected at the checkpoint, causing a potential cancer to stop dead in its tracks.

Recently, Loros's research team found that cell damage can trigger the body's biological clock to reset itself. She suspects that protective proteins might fool these cells into thinking they're at the time in their cycle when cell division doesn't occur, thus averting cancer in the making.

Bottom line: Can fiber prevent cancer?

Technically, no. But eat it anyway. We'll explain. Several years ago, a pair of studies suggested that dietary fiber could reduce the risk of colon cancer. But a new review of 13 studies encompassing 725,628 people in the *Journal of the American Medical Association* found no such connection.

Researchers believe the discrepancy lies in the fact that people who eat fiber tend also to take multivitamins, limit red meats, and consume folate-rich foods, all of which have been shown to reduce the risk of cancer in the first 5 feet of the large intestine (i.e., your colon). Fiber alone, however, "won't affect your colon-cancer risk one way or the other," says John Baron, MD, a professor of medicine at Dartmouth Medical School. What it will do is cut your risk of getting cancer in your rectum (the last 8 to 10 inches of said intestine).

The same *JAMA* review found that eating 25 grams of fiber per day lowers rectal-cancer risk by 15 percent. Why the difference between the two ends of the intestine? Doctor's aren't sure. But what is clear is that there are many benefits to dietary fiber, from improving regularity to preventing heart disease. The best way to get 25 grams: Eat whole foods, like oatmeal (4 grams per cup), blackberries (7.6 grams), and split-pea soup (16.3 grams).

My freckles are multiplying. Should I worry?

Yes, says *Men's Health* dermatology advisor John F. Romano, MD. Freckles are a sign of sun damage. They turn up after prolonged sun exposure but often fade until you're in the sun again. Freckles aren't precancerous, but they are a warning to limit your time in the sun and use plenty of sunscreen. If you have lots of freckles and are over the age of 30, arrange checkups by a dermatologist every 2 or 3 years.

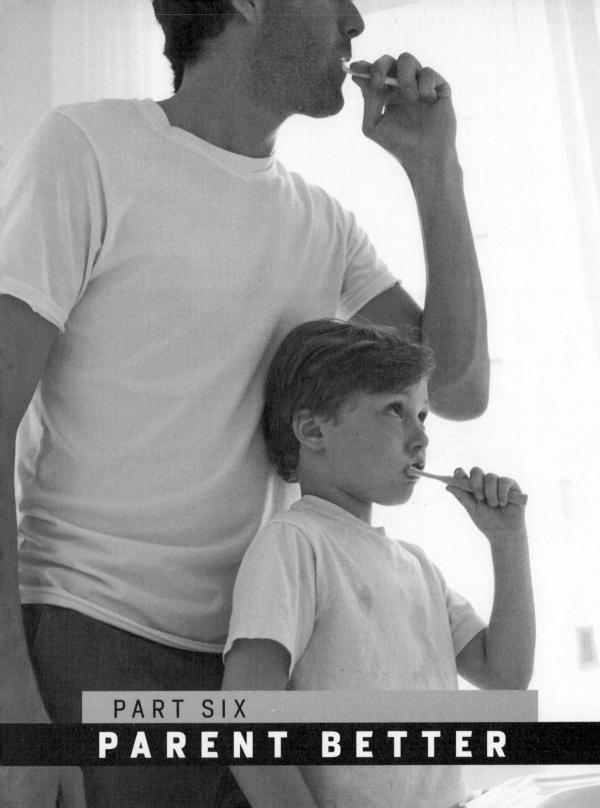

PART SIX

PARENT BETTER

MORE THAN JUST THE UGLY MOM

HEED THESE REVELATIONS FROM A 21ST-CENTURY SUPERDAD

BY RICH MALOOF

I have cooked pasta shaped like rabbits, and all my shirt shoulders are stained with spit-up. I can change diapers with one hand and sing my kid to sleep. I know the difference between a onesie, a binky, and a boppie. And the theme to *Elmo's World* is stuck in my head where a Foo Fighters riff should be. I am a 21st-century father. Have mercy on me.

New dads take on more than we ever saw our fathers do. We're bread-winners and cooks, coaches and bottle washers. Like creatures that have crawled out of the Galapagos waters for the very first time, we're out of our element and frankly a little confused. Here's what parenting looks like from this side of the changing table.

THERE'S NO ROAD MAP

I'm a reasonably secure male, but I confess to feeling a little less virile on days when I take my 3-year-old son, Daniel, to preschool near our home in Brooklyn, New York, and pass a stream of guys in suits headed the other way, toward Wall Street. Pushing a stroller in lockstep with the moms and singing nursery rhymes, it's tough to fight the feeling that I left my gonads back home in a jar.

PERCENTAGE OF MEN WHO SAY HEATHCLIFF HUXTABLE (BILL COSBY ON *THE COSBY SHOW*) IS THE IDEAL TV DAD:

49

One recent day on the way to school, I had also tucked Danny's 3-month-old sister, Tess, into the back of our wildly overpriced double stroller. She burst into tears along the way, so I picked her up and held her close to me. That's when she started grabbing for my shirt as if she thought I had a breast full of milk under there. And why shouldn't she think so? She doesn't even technically need a dad yet. As far as Tess can tell, I'm just the ugly mom.

Which gets to the crux of the issue for me. Before our generation, the roles of moms and dads had been in place for centuries. Our parents lived a domesticated version of what had existed since time immemorial: Mothers made the home comfortable and raised the kids while fathers went out and chased dinner around with a rock. I have an excellent dad, but I can't remember him ever handing me a sandwich in a Ziploc and reminding me not to poop in my Spider-Man undies.

Sticking to established roles may not have done much for equality, but it did make things simple. A man knew who he was and what he was expected to do. Picture your father wearing a Baby Björn and scanning the pharmacy shelves for nipple pads and you'll understand what I'm talking about. It's completely different today. Now guys have to negotiate roles with our wives and try to come up with some balance of work life, home life, and sanity. We want to put roofs over our families' heads, but we also want to spend more time under them.

Like a lot of new dads, I can intellectualize my way into being at ease with this contemporary division of responsibilities. But it's a tough balance to strike. When my wife, Kris, recently said she was ready to go back to work, I told her I didn't need any help taking care of things at home. Cleaning up the kitchen the next evening, I then complained that I had to do all of my stuff and half of hers. Oops. It's as if my progressive thinking about sharing responsibilities has evolved ahead of my natural inclination to protect and provide. Fortunately, Kris and I don't throw things at each other with children in the house.

BENEATH THE DIAPER

When Danny was a newborn, I didn't give much thought to his gender—he was a baby first, a boy second. Not until a sparkling arc of urine hit me in the neck as I was changing him did I start to consider the difference between parenting boys and girls. Now that we have one of each, I realize I'm hard-pressed to treat them exactly the same way.

My armchair theory is that men have more baggage with boys. We can't help but imagine them as little versions of ourselves, and with that comes the need to make them better men than we are. In our sons we see our own untapped potential, so we constantly direct and correct them. I want my son to write the great American novel, travel more than I have, and play guitar at Madison Square Garden. I know the poor little guy is still working on the alphabet, but it's difficult to resist being meddlesome. He must find me very annoying.

Girls we don't expect to understand. We've learned this from experience, having spent years stymied by stuff like why you enjoy TV shows that make you cry. So we're free to lavish our daughters with affection and protection. In fact, as I write this I'm awaiting the arrival of the hermetically sealed tube my daughter will live in until she's 26 and ready to date.

THIS IS EVOLUTION?

A 2000 study published in the journal *Evolution and Human Behavior* found that new fathers experience sympathetic hormonal changes after the birth of a child, including a drop in testosterone levels. This is not only alarming but ridiculously inconvenient. Here we've been summoned to our primal role as Chief Protector, and the well of masculinity is going dry. We're supposed to be keeping the bear from the cave entrance, but instead we're inside humming lullabies.

Thing is, after a lifetime of measuring our sensitivity in teaspoons, having kids turns us to mush. Like Superman brought to his knees by a fragment of his home planet, we crumble when we see a tiny bit of ourselves staring back at us. That's love, and that's great, but it comes with a dose of vulnerability and defensiveness we didn't bargain for.

NUMBER OF YEARS YOUNGER HAVING 1 TO 3 KIDS CAN MAKE YOU LOOK:

2

Those parents who pick fights at school hockey games? I always thought they were nuts. But the first time somebody fouls my kid in a game, I'll have to be fitted for a straitjacket.

The other day, I spotted another dad stumbling his way through the Galapagos of new dad-hood. He was out for a run with his kid, explaining the Walk/Don't Walk signs while pushing a jogging stroller with one hand and— I kid you not—balancing a pizza box with the other. All at once he was being a parent and teacher, promoting his own survival, and quite literally putting dinner on the table. I recognized his expression: a mixture of pride, bewilderment, and determination. A little lost without a map, but trying like hell to be a good dad. And, no, he's not going to ask for directions.

MY UNEXPECTED CHILDREN

WHEN I LOST MY BEST FRIEND, I GAINED RESPONSIBILITY
FOR HIS FAMILY. AND MY LIFE IS ALL THE RICHER

BY HARLAN COBEN

When I woke up that horrible morning, the lead photo on my Internet home page showed a small plane crash. I didn't think much about it; it had gone down in someplace called Kirksville, Missouri—someplace I'd never heard of. I live in the New Jersey suburbs, outside New York City. The only reason the story had made that front screen at all was that "miraculously" there had been at least two survivors.

But 3 hours later, I'd learn that my dear friend Steve Miller had been on that flight. And 5 hours later, I'd be at his New York City town house with a telephone pressed to my ear, my heart pounding with a slow thud, as family and friends sat silent in the next room, waiting for the American Airlines employee to confirm our worst fear: Yes, there had been two survivors from the crash of Flight 5966. But Dr. Steven Z. Miller wasn't one of them.

Steve was magic. We have a habit of raising those who die prematurely to saintlike status, but Steve was so beloved, so accomplished, that he always made you feel a little wanting. He was an internationally renowned physician, teacher, and director of pediatric emergency medicine at Columbia's New York–Presbyterian Hospital. The medical students of the prestigious Columbia University College of Physicians and Surgeons had voted him Teacher of the Year the past 5 years running.

Everyone loved Steve. He was genuine and smart and talented. He was decisive at work, neurotic and insecure at home, endearing everywhere. I had no better friend.

Steve was the least judgmental guy I knew. He asked questions and genuinely cared about the answers. I flash back more than a decade: My first Myron Bolitar novel, *Deal Breaker*, a small-print-run paperback, is just about to be published to absolutely no acclaim or fanfare. Yet Steve has demanded an advance copy. He doesn't just read it; he studies it as if it is the Talmud. We meet up with our families in a park near Coronado Beach in San Diego. He has the book with him. We sit on the grass, and he starts peppering me with detailed questions about motivations and character and plot twists. We sit like that in the sun for a very long time, and I love every minute of it. And I can't believe—still can't believe—that we won't do it again.

I flash back to a more recent time, a Springsteen concert at Giants Stadium. It's pouring, and we're on our feet, drenched. The rain has plastered Steve's long gray locks to his face. He is standing behind his wife, Dodi, rocking back and forth. We're screaming the lyrics, two guys in our forties, lost in the bliss of this release. Our eyes meet, and we give each other the smallest of nods, and we just know. We know it is one of those moments that both of us will always remember; that we'll be able to take it out on a dark day, and it will make us smile.

I have lived a life of few regrets. But I regret that I didn't see Steve enough. We had talked about a trip to Argentina, his clan and mine. I bagged it because the flight was too long. That pang never goes away. So if nothing else, if you've read enough of this article already, call that one friend because it's been too long since you had a beer with him. Do it now.

But this isn't a eulogy.

When that plane crashed on October 19, 2004, I knew that New York–Presbyterian had lost its best doctor, that the underserved patients of Washington Heights would be forever shortchanged, that Dodi had lost the man of her dreams, that his three children—Jesse, nearly 12; Maya, 11; and Nico, only 6—had lost a father, but because I am a typical guy, I was worried about missing my friend.

So I, as a man, as a friend, decided to do what I could. It was partly out of obligation, partly out of guilt, and partly—maybe mostly—out of selfishness.

I couldn't let Steve go.

But this is what you start with, this feeling of obligation. You want— no, need—to help in some way. You want to make the path somehow easier for Dodi, Jesse, Maya, and Nico—but mostly, you do it to hold on to your friend a little longer. You can't be with him anymore, can't catch that flick you kept saying you were going to catch, can't go to that game, or—to get heavier—share life's successes and disappointments. But maybe, just maybe, you can still do something for your friend and thus be with him.

> **PERCENTAGE OF MEN WHO SAY THEY'RE A BETTER FATHER THAN THEIR FATHER WAS:**
> **61**

It started slowly. Jesse and Maya are sports fans. We went to Madison Square Garden and checked out a few games. It was always a blast, but after I dropped them back at the house, it would be as if I were waiting to tell Steve about it, as if I could still share it with him and maybe get his nod of approval.

It kept going on. One morning, we went to the taping of one of Jesse's favorite shows on ESPN. They drove out to our house and played in our yard. We visited them and walked through the city. One night, about a month after Steve's death, Jesse instant-messaged me on the computer. We chatted that way for a while. Then his sister Maya did the same. I started looking for them on my buddy list. I still do. We talk about nothing, about school, about how Mom is doing, that kind of thing.

On December 10, 2005, a little more than a year after the plane crash, Jesse Miller was called to the Torah for his bar mitzvah. Looking up at him from my seat with the congregation, I saw Steve, of course. But as his beautiful son ended the service by singing "Imagine" by John Lennon, I realized something simple and profound.

I love Jesse.

I love Jesse and Maya and Nico. Not because I have to. Not in the way we love/tolerate our friends' kids. I love them in a way that I love no other children but my own. I love them in a fierce way. I will never let anyone hurt them. I will protect them. I will make sure that they get what they need. If they are in trouble, I will rush to their side. Always.

It is not as a father figure, not even a substitute or part-time one. It is something different, something deep and profound and unexpected. Doing things with Steve's family is no longer a manly obligation, if it ever really was. It has become something that I want to do, that I really look forward to doing.

Steve spent his last New Year's Eve at my home—his family and mine in a rather placid sleepover. I have two pictures in my office from that day—one of Steve, Dodi, and their three kids in goofy "2004" glasses, another of Steve and me in our pajamas after getting doused with Silly String. I treasure those pictures more than I can express.

So this past December, our two families decide to get together for New Year's again, without Steve. With our goofy "2006" glasses packed in a suitcase, we drive up to New Hampshire to spend the weekend on a farm. Milking cows, gathering eggs, going on a hayride—Steve, the neurotic city boy, would have hated it. We all laugh about that.

But we take two cars. Jesse, now 13, sits next to me. We've brought our iPods. We play songs for each other. We sing along. We shout out a version of Elton John's "Levon" that is so bad, I feel as though I need to write Elton a letter of apology. Jesse asks me questions and genuinely cares about the answers. So like Steve. It is bittersweet, but it is better.

I hear the echo of my dead friend in his son. I drive, steering with my wrists, and we both sing.

I feel Steve, and part of me wants to cry, but another part of me—a much larger part of me—just wants to hear his son keep singing.

PUSHED AWAY

AN INSIDIOUS BRAINWASHING CAN DESTROY THE
ONCE-CLOSE RELATIONSHIPS OF CHILDREN AND THEIR
DIVORCED DADS. SOME PSYCHOLOGISTS CALL IT "PARENTAL
ALIENATION SYNDROME." FATHERS CALL IT THEIR WORST
NIGHTMARE. READ ON TO KEEP IT FROM BECOMING YOURS

BY JOHN SEDGWICK

Jeff Opperman, a 49-year-old corporate-communications officer in Seymour, Connecticut, got the first gut-churning clue of how ruinous his
divorce was going to be to his relationship with his younger son the
night it became clear he and his wife, Anne, had to part.

They'd been married for 17 years, but it hadn't been going well. "We
were fighting and drifting apart," says Opperman, "and the more we
fought, the more we drifted apart, and the more we drifted apart, the
more we fought." They decided to hold off telling Alec, just 11, until he'd
finished camp that summer. But the marriage was so rocky that Jeff
and Anne arrived in separate cars to take him home, leaving it to Alec
to choose which car to ride home in. He picked his mother's—a fateful
choice, as things turned out. "God knows what she said to him in that
car for an hour and a half," Opperman says.

The next night, when he and Anne "got into it" in their bedroom, she
burst out the door and raced down to Alec's room, where she yelled,
Opperman recalls, "the most horrid, disgraceful things, calling me a
liar, a cheat, a son of a bitch, just everything." Tears streamed down
Alec's reddened face, but he didn't try to defend his dad. Instead, to
Opperman's astonishment, he started to chime in, feebly parroting some
of his mother's charges, even though he'd always been close to his father.
When Opperman tried to give the boy a reassuring hug, Anne abruptly
stepped between them and, claiming that Jeff was going to hurt the
boy, threatened to call the police if he came any closer. Opperman

backed off, not wanting to risk a bigger scene in front of his son. "Alec cried his eyes out," Opperman recalls. "Just cried and cried."

That was 6 years ago, but it established the dynamic by which Jeff became the designated ogre parent and Alec became Anne's exclusive possession. Jeff acknowledges that he hadn't been a perfect husband. "When a marriage breaks down, both parties are at fault, and ours was no different," he says. But regardless of who was responsible for the divorce, Jeff feels his ex should have protected Alec from the negative aspects of the relationship. Instead, he claims, she burdened their son with her pain and sense of betrayal—and Alec responded by aligning himself fully with his mother and emotionally cutting off his dad.

Although Opperman was granted joint custody and lives just 10 minutes away, he has since seen his son only for the briefest intervals—despite repeatedly taking his ex to court over custody violations. "The court adopts this tough-talking John Wayne attitude," Opperman recounts. "'You will take the child to counseling. You will allow the child to maintain relations with the father. You will, you will, you will.' But my ex doesn't do any of it—and nothing happens." Despite all Opperman's efforts, the court has been both reluctant to force Alec to spend time with a father he wants nothing to do with and unwilling to compel Alec's mother by threat of jail time.

All this leaves Opperman out in the cold. His Christmas and birthday presents to Alec go unacknowledged. When Opperman calls, Alec will occasionally pick up, but when he hears that it's his father on the line, he won't speak. All Jeff hears is Alec's breath in the receiver before he sets the phone down. Last summer, Opperman came to the house to pick up his older son, Alec's brother. There were lights on in Alec's bedroom, and Opperman could see the back of Alec's head as he stared at a computer screen. Jeff honked the horn, hoping to get Alec's attention. "I was sure he could hear me," Jeff recalls. "But Alec never even turned his head."

Opperman's desperation is hardly unique. About 40 percent of children living with their mothers don't see their fathers so much as once a year. Even allowing for fathers who are at war, in prison, or otherwise unavailable, statistics like that force the question: Are there really that many men out there who simply don't care about their kids and vice versa? Or is something more sinister at work?

WHY FATHERS GET TURNED AWAY

Nightmarish as the tale of Alec's transformation may sound, it is not an entirely uncommon experience for divorced parents to witness this change in their children, and a new term is entering the psychiatric lexicon to describe it: Parental Alienation Syndrome, or PAS. "I see it all the time," says Lynn McNeese Swank, a Jonesboro, Georgia, lawyer specializing in custody issues. "A child is manipulated by one parent or the other on a subconscious basis—the survival level, really—fundamentally altering his understanding of reality. It can take years to undo, if it ever is at all."

And the damage can be extensive. Now 43, Peter G., of Houston, says he's still not over the fact that his mother alienated him from his father; it created overwhelming "trust issues" that have kept him from forming any serious romantic attachments. The alienation started abruptly one afternoon, when he was 13. His mother, who'd won sole custody of all eight children, herded the kids into her psychotherapist's office and, apparently with the therapist's blessing, had each one complete the sentence: "I hate my dad because . . ." Peter could tell that his mother had coached some of the children on what to say because they echoed her own words about how their father had "abandoned" the family and was, as she often implied, a "no-good philandering bastard" besides. But Peter clung to the memories of happy days he'd spent with his father working on the family car. He fled the room in tears along with another brother who felt the same way. And that created a permanent family divide between the kids who followed Mom and the two outcasts who still felt some sympathy for Dad. "My mom was the saint, and my dad was the devil," Peter says. "That was her line. And if I didn't agree with that, then obviously I had 'unresolved issues.'"

The pressure from his mother and siblings to turn against his father was unrelenting. "Every day was a battle," Peter recalls. "I felt like a soldier going back and back and back to a war that never ends."

In his despair, he turned to drugs and fell in with the "wrong people."

The father didn't respond well to this merciless ostracization campaign against him, either. He suffered a nervous breakdown—seemingly confirming his deficiency as a parent. Later, Peter discovered that, while his father had indeed been unfaithful, his mother was the far more shameless philanderer, having had a number of wildly inappropriate affairs. "That's when I realized my mom was total bullshit. She ran me out of the family to make sure her secrets got kept." Concludes Peter: "Basically, I felt I had no parents at all. Which one could I trust?"

That, of course, is the cruelty of parental alienation. It's *Sophie's Choice* in reverse: A child has to choose between his parents, consigning one or the other to emotional oblivion. "A child shouldn't have to choose," says another grown-up PAS child, 27-year-old Christine L., showing a flash of anger in discussing what must have been a tortured childhood. In her case, it was her dad who had custody and who pushed her mother completely out of their children's lives. "It's so selfish on the part of the alienating parent. It helps him deal with the pain, but it just burdens the child with it," says Christine.

EMOTIONAL EXILE AND LEGAL LIMBO

Explosive as PAS is, the phenomenon continues to fly largely below the radar, until a high-profile case kicks it into public awareness, as happened recently when newspapers reported that actor Alec Baldwin accused his ex, Kim Basinger, of turning their 10-year-old daughter Ireland against him.

Strictly speaking, PAS occurs when impressionable young children join forces with one parent against the other, often attended by the "in" parent's deliberate thwarting of any contact with the children by the "out" one, no matter what the courts might officially require in terms of custody or visitation. Classically, the alienation is perpetrated by the wife against the husband, although both parents are fully capable of it if they are sufficiently desperate—and venomous. "It's a terrible act of cruelty," says clinical psychologist Richard A. Warshak, PhD, a leading scholar of the disorder who has written a book, *Divorce Poison*, describing the condition of PAS. To him, the behavior is reminiscent of the brainwashing by religious cults but with this difference: Cults affect a relatively small number of Americans. With close to half of all marriages ending in divorce and a vast majority of them involving children, the number of children at risk for PAS, he says, runs well into the millions.

"Whatever their intentions, these parents are stealing their children's souls," Dr. Warshak contends. "They are rendering them incapable of receiving love from the people who have the most love to give them." Some of the alienating behavior is simply petty, like deriding an ex-husband's cooking skills or housekeeping so the children will think less of him; or it can be insidious, like encouraging the children to call the alienated father by his first name, diminishing his stature.

Some of the alienating techniques are simple propaganda, similar to what combatants use in wartime, Dr. Warshak says. "You repeat negative messages until they are so deeply imbedded in memory, the child doesn't really know how he's come to know them." One father saw his youngest daughter, just 8, at a meeting attended by an array of attorneys and psychologists to appraise their relationship, write on a whiteboard, "Dad, you are an asshole." Only she spelled the word "asswhole," since she was obviously unfamiliar with the term. For good measure, the girl added, "And you're a suck-up," another word that was not likely part of her vocabulary. She wrapped up with a strangely adult send-off: "I never want to see you again."

Alienating parents have been known to clip the heads off their ex-spouses' photos in family albums, deliberately lose their letters or telephone messages, treat them like nonpeople at events like a kid's soccer game, or, in one case, mount a photograph of the ex on a dartboard for family target practice. And it is not just the father who is alienated. Everything about him can be relegated to the discard pile—his side of the family, his associations, his friends, even the family dog, if it is considered to have been primarily his. "It's tribal warfare," says Dr. Warshak. "Anything associated with the alienated parent is tainted and has to be rejected." McNeese Swank said one mother insisted that her son change his clothes before he visited his dad's house and then leave those garments there, lest they somehow contaminate her own house if he were to bring them back.

Some of the alienating verbiage is more like a political attack ad that, Dr. Warshak says, "draws attention to the problems of your opponent, while talking only positively about yourself." A mother might be braiding her daughter's hair, he says, and ask pointedly, "Does Daddy do that for you?" The implication, of course, is that Daddy doesn't—because he doesn't care.

Fathers used to playing the role of disciplinarian can lose points with their young children for encouraging a masculine-style toughness and adherence to rules, and mothers win them for being indulgent and cozy. A wholesaler named Richard Burke lost out to his ex when he insisted that their two children go to a stricter private school than the one attended by their friends. "My wife told them," he reports, "'It's really a shame that Dad makes you go to that hard school where you have to wear a uniform and do all that homework.'" She also bought them cell phones and in-bedroom satellite TV. Before long, the kids opted out of the school and moved in full-time with Mom. The son was the first to go. When he refused to come out of his mother's house to go for his usual nights at his father's, Burke called the police. He showed them the custody agreement and pointed to the calendar. "See? This is my day," he insisted. But it was no use. "The police didn't want to get into the middle of it. They said, 'Yeah, but the kid doesn't want to go.' And that was the end of it." The sister later repeated the same scenario. And the courts offered Burke no support. "They just don't understand what parental alienation is when they're looking right at it," Burke sighs.

"Getting custody is like getting a judgment in small-claims court," says Reena Sommer, PhD, a divorce-and-custody consultant in Galveston, Texas. "You still gotta go collect." Adds psychotherapist J. Michael Bone, PhD, a leading authority on PAS, "Court orders are ignored all the time. When a father objects, a judge will say, 'What am I supposed to do? Throw the mother in jail?' You may have to go back multiple times to get visitation rights enforced, and it can take months. By then, the child can be more alienated than ever."

THE TOLL ON THE CHILDREN

The legacy of such warfare on the alienated children, Dr. Warshak says, is terrible and lasting—depression, low self-esteem, and strained relationships for decades to come.

"Alienated children are like ghosts," says Timothy Hoffman, PhD, a Massachusetts family therapist who has treated many of these kids. "They don't fully exist, because they are trapped between two adults who are battling to be right. Allegiance, betrayal, deciding whom to believe—it's a dreadful position for a child to be in." In later life, Dr. Hoffman goes on, these alienated children are likely to struggle to develop trusting relationships, to be emotionally shut down, and to be prone to an identity crisis after ultimately discovering the truth about an alienating parent. "They may find they've aligned themselves with a parent who styled himself or herself as the victim but then turns out to be the perpetrator," says Dr. Hoffman. "What a betrayal that can be."

For the alienated parent, the brutality of the experience is often intensified by the nuclear bomb of custody disputes—a charge of physical or sexual abuse coming straight from the child's mouth on some witness stand or in a court-appointed therapist's office. Many PAS experts agree that the syndrome is sometimes used to cover up real abuse; and because 79 percent of confirmed abuse cases involve a parent as the abuser, the courts have a hard time distinguishing between situations involving actual abuse and allegations that are the result of PAS. But since nothing asserts, or provokes, a child's alienation quite like charges of abuse, they are a regular feature of PAS cases.

"The parent who files the charges is automatically given protection," says Burt W., a 48-year-old chemical engineer from Virginia, whose ex-wife orchestrated his two daughters' claims that he'd molested them in the shower. (The court later ruled there was no evidence to substantiate the claims.) The accuser rarely has to submit to the polygraph tests or psychiatric evaluations that are imposed on the defendant. "But the other person is damaged, isolated, and completely powerless. You want my advice? Learn to manage your anger, or it will eat you alive. Me, I was pumping weights like never before, and I was still driving up to hilltops to scream my lungs out," says Burt.

THE SUDDEN EXPLOSION OF ALIENATION

It was the psychologist Richard Gardner, MD, who first identified Parental Alienation Syndrome in 1985 after he began to notice an increase in children of divorce who seemed to have it in for their dads

⏩ALIENATION ALERT

Here are some warnings signs your ex may be turning the kids against you.

⏩ Your child starts to talk about you and your ex in black-and-white terms. He might say, "You always try to embarrass me. Mom would never do that."

⏩ Your kid refers to the divorce as "when you left us," which means he may be parroting your ex-wife's emotions and even her words. Another: "You're trying to buy my love with toys."

⏩ You taught your son to play soccer, but he quits. If this is part of a pattern, it may indicate he's rejecting things associated with you.

⏩ He starts calling you by your first name, indicating that you no longer warrant the respect due a parent.

⏩ While looking at a happy father-child photograph, your kid says, "I was smiling because you told me to." His mother could be reinterpreting old memories for him.

for no good reason. In all but 10 percent of cases, he wrote in 1987, the mother was the alienating parent and the father the "target parent" with the bull's-eye on his back. In his book *Parental Alienation Syndrome and the Differentiation Between Fabricated and Genuine Child Sex Abuse*, Dr. Gardner, who died in 2001, attributed the behavior to a combination of maternal entitlement and a custodial privilege that had traditionally won mothers special influence over their children—and thus the means and incentive to turn them against their fathers should that primacy be threatened.

And it was starting to be threatened, for this was the era when custody standards were shifting because of a reappraisal of parental sex roles. The "tender years presumption" by which children had long been routinely awarded to mothers had been evolving since the 1970s into a "best interests of the child presumption" that was more open to giving custody to fathers. The battle for the children was on, and, as Dr. Gardner told it, some mothers went ruthlessly on the attack to win over the children they considered rightfully theirs. The mothers drove the anti-Dad messages in deep, turning the children into the chief accusers of the fathers they once loved. But Dr. Gardner noted a "rehearsed quality to the speech" and suspiciously adult "phraseology." He noticed that small children might claim Dad "harasses us." But the evidence they gave was often slim. "He always used to say to me, 'Don't interrupt,'" one child complained. Said another: "He always used to speak very loud when he told me to brush my teeth."

While the term was intended to be merely descriptive, the designation Parental Alienation Syndrome soon was seized upon by lawyers as a way for aggrieved dads to fight back. But the designation of PAS is still caught in the crosswinds between psychology and the law, with lawyers eager to make use of a tactic that has such a powerfully effective medical overlay and psychologists reluctant to confer a definitive diagnosis on a fairly blurry cluster of behaviors. "PAS is hard to accept without clear, objective markers," says Robert E. Emery, PhD, a psychologist at the University of Virginia who has written critically of the syndrome. He notes that PAS has not been accepted in the *Diagnostic and Statistical Manual of Mental Disorders*—Fourth Edition (or *DSM-IV*), the bible of accepted psychiatric disorders. (Neither have such commonly accepted phenomena as Stockholm Syndrome, for example, in which people held hostage for extended periods come to sympathize with their captors.) Defenders point out that there can be a long lag before new diagnoses are recognized. To Dr. Emery, PAS is simply too much in the eye of the beholder. "Expert A will say it is," he says, "but Expert B will say it isn't."

A lot of the dispute is simply over the terminology. Few psychologists doubt that one parent could turn a child against the other if she put her mind to it. "In developmental psychology, we know that kids can be manipulated to hate and fear others," says Dr. Warshak. "It's absurd to think that can't happen in a divorce situation." After all, adds Dr. Bone, the litigation process encourages it. "The child is already being taught that he has been abandoned by one parent," Dr. Bone says. "He is not going to risk being abandoned by the other." So he will exhibit unquestioning loyalty to the parent who is brainwashing him because the child is terrified of being abandoned again and becoming a virtual orphan. Hence the pathological extremes of love and hate that mark the alienated child, who sees nothing but good in the alienator and nothing but bad

⏩HOW TO FIGHT BACK

Once you were close; now your child treats you like a criminal and takes his mother's side in every dispute. It's tempting to fire back at your ex—to tell your side of the story to your child, defend yourself, put the blame where you think it belongs. But that's not going to help—in fact, it will only hurt both your child and your relationship with him. Instead, follow these guidelines.

Make your house a safe haven: Parents who have retained access to their kids have had success by offering their children a sanctuary from the vilification, making it a point never to bad-mouth the other spouse in their child's presence, no matter how much bile is coming from the other side. An alienated father named Kevin Askew maintained that policy, and he could see his son grow more comfortable with him by the hour. "At my house," he says, "my son could be a little boy and just play."

Talk to intermediaries: Reach out to your children's teachers, religious leaders, or coaches, says attorney Lynn McNeese Swank. "A teacher or someone might be able to tell the kid, 'You know, Dad isn't so bad as you think.'" Fathers we've spoken with have battled the alienation by joining the PTA, coaching the kids' sports teams, or organizing Indian Princess meetings. This also allows you to be around your children's friends, who might decide that Dad is actually kind of cool.

Expect respect: If your child starts calling you by your first name or labeling you in some way, immediately state that such behavior will not be tolerated, and explain that you disapprove of pejorative labels of all sorts.

Be empathetic: If your child repeats something negative his mother has said about you, reply that it must be difficult for the child to hear such things and that even parents, when they get angry, say things they shouldn't. Explain that no matter what his mom might say, no one is entirely good or entirely bad. If your ex tells the child a lie about you, simply say, "Mom's mistaken about that."

Don't give up: As painful as the situation may be for you now, children grow up, and one day they'll figure out the truth for themselves. If you withdraw, you lose. Stay involved.

in the target parent. And, says McNeese Swank, that fear is likely to be all the stronger if the alienating parent is the mom: "Ninety percent of the time, she's the one thing they have to look to for shelter, sustenance, and support." Indeed, the fear etched on the alienated child's face is one of the hallmarks of the disorder. The Virginia chemical engineer, Burt W., saw the look on one of his daughters when he was finally allowed to see her after the mother had created that elaborate molestation charge against him. Not long before, the girl had performed circus acts with Burt, balancing upside down on his knees on the living-room floor. Now she was, he said, "standoffish, wary, like she was frightened of me."

UNDOING THE DAMAGE

Because alienated children aren't allowed to establish a rapport with their noncustodial parent, it can be a stunning surprise to a child to finally encounter the truth about a father who had long been vilified. Edward C., a 49-year-old computer programmer, was so alienated by his wife that she withheld custody of his daughter even from the grave. Dying of cancer, she entrusted their daughter to her aunt as legal guardian and to the in-laws of her son by a previous marriage. Because of everything the mother had told the daughter about her dad, the girl was reluctant to get in touch with him. But on a lark, she sent her dad a Father's Day card and called him 2 months later. Soon thereafter, Edward took her shopping for school clothes and out for an afternoon of horseback riding. "I loved it," the girl told the in-laws, amazed. "He was so nice!" To this day, they remain close. "With my ex-wife, all love was conditional," Edward says. "If my daughter did it the way my ex wanted, she'd love her. If not, she'd rage at her or give her the silent treatment. It was completely controlling."

Happily, as in Edward's case, the alienation can end eventually, although experts say a final reconciliation is far from guaranteed—for the simple reason that the alienating parent cannot keep total mind control over the children forever. They grow up, leave the house where all the secrets are kept, and eventually come to discover the truth. Difficult as it can be, alienated parents need to maintain a positive, welcoming attitude for the day the phone finally rings.

It can be a long, anxious wait. Despite his best efforts to stay in touch with his children, Burke—the wholesaler whose custody agreement the police refused to enforce—hasn't seen his son in 3 years. That left Burke stumped as to how to acknowledge the boy's 18th birthday. In desperation, Burke decided on an extreme measure. He hired a small plane to fly a banner over the school, wishing his son a happy 18th birthday and signed "I LOVE YOU, DAD," all in huge block letters. Through the grapevine, Burke learned that his son's friends thought the banner was "great." And his son?

"I haven't heard a word."

GENERATION XXL

SEVEN WAYS TO REFORM AMERICA'S PHYSICAL EDUCATION—AND TRANSFORM KIDS FROM FAT TO FIT

BY SCOTT QUILL

Taking whole milk out of schools won't make kids thinner. Neither will levying taxes on video games. These are actual proposals—by the Illinois State Board of Education and the New York Legislature, no less. But they're misguided, arising predictably from misinformation.

You don't need to be told that American kids are getting fatter. You've seen the evidence waddling toward you in the mall.

What we all could use instead is a clear-eyed look at the situation, minus the panic: How bad is it, how'd we get here, and what are we going to do about it? That's where *Men's Health* can help. We've read the research and talked to the top experts. We've visited schools and spoken with teachers, coaches, and kids. And we've gotten as close to the truth as we can.

Most kids don't know the truth. Politically correct words—"heavyset," "husky"—make denial easier for everyone, and loose fashions disguise flab. Misleading measurements such as body-mass index (BMI) greatly underestimate the number of overweight children.

"Kids who would have been called overweight 15 to 20 years ago are now considered husky," says David Watson, MD, a pediatrician who works with schools in Massachusetts. "Moderately overweight kids now see themselves as being normal weight."

There's denial about levels of physical activity, too. Hard research busts us, adults and children alike, for claiming to be more active than we are.

The ultimate result: We're shortening our children's lives. A study in the *New England Journal of Medicine* reports that our kids' life spans are expected to be 2 to 5 years shorter than our own—because of fat. And

PERCENTAGE OF SCHOOLS THAT MEET NATIONALLY RECOMMENDED EXERCISE REQUIREMENTS:

8

the time they will have may be plagued by problems. More than 9 million overweight children are predisposed to depression, negative self-image, high blood pressure, stroke, and diabetes.

In our research, we found hope—the start of something exciting. We found it in places like Hartland, Wisconsin, in 18-year-old Corey Wise, a recent graduate of Arrowhead Union High School. Three years ago, Wise was a fat, slothful sophomore, suspended after two failing grades. Then he found Club Arrowhead, his school's new physical-education course. It's almost a health club for teenagers, not the lap-running, square-dancing classes that failed today's adults.

Corey's 225 pounds seemed to morph from fat to muscle and migrated from his belly to his chest, shoulders, and arms. As his body-fat percentage dropped, his grade-point average rose—from 1.9 to 3.0. (See "How Exercise Makes Your Child Smarter," on page 240.)

But while Arrowhead may be the future of physical education, and a number of schools across the country are revamping their phys-ed programs, most remain clueless.

That's why we culled the secrets of America's fittest schools and asked experts to help create a curriculum to rebuild any student body. On the following pages, you'll find our prescription for saving a generation, and it's your responsibility to help.

FOCUS ON FIRST GRADERS

A student who enters high school overweight has only a slight chance of reaching a normal weight by adulthood, report researchers at Baylor College of Medicine in Waco, Texas, who studied more than 800 people, at age 10 and again between the ages of 19 and 35. High-school freshmen at healthy weights, on the other hand, are four times as likely to stay slim as adults.

It's important to hook them early. "By the time kids reach the third grade, they're making excuses for why they don't participate in exercise," says Jim Liston, CSCS, owner of Catz Competitive Athlete Training Zone, in Pasadena, California. Encouraging them in the early grades is crucial, he says. "There's no fear of failure in kindergartners and first graders, but somewhere between first and third, kids become conscious of their bodies and of what other people think."

If they give up on sports, "it really classifies them as outsiders," adds Dr. Watson, "particularly the boys, because athleticism defines the maleness of an American elementary or middle schooler."

FACT: Fat kids often stay fat.

PRESCRIPTION: Schedule vigorous play throughout the early grades.

LIFT THEIR SPIRITS

Overweight kids prefer lifting weights to aerobic activity, according to a report by the National Strength and Conditioning Association. That's mainly because they can lift more weight than their lighter peers can, and endurance isn't as much of a factor.

"In every study I've seen on young children, the only workouts that have changed body composition include some type of strength exercise," says Wayne Westcott, PhD, author of the report. "Once kids develop strength and a higher metabolic rate, they can enjoy activity and burn calories."

Realizing you're stronger is an instant confidence boost, as Arrowhead junior Anders Rahm can attest. He has asthma and Osgood-Schlatter disease (the patellar tendons pull away from the shinbone). A strength and flexibility course called Zero Hour—held before school—helped alleviate Rahm's pain while improving endurance and helping him pack on 15 pounds of muscle.

FACT: Weight lifting burns calories, changes bodies, and builds confidence.

PRESCRIPTION: Make strength training available.

FIND THE EXPERTS OUTSIDE (AND INSIDE) THE SCHOOL

America's best trainers work with professional athletes to shave their 40-yard-dash times. Of course, they won't come to your high school's track. Not if you don't ask, that is.

Arrowhead's activities director, Geoff Steinbach, sought out world-renowned speed coach Loren Seagrave, whom he knew from the University of Wisconsin. Seagrave helped develop the concept for Club Arrowhead and returns frequently to teach a class at the school. Then Steinbach looked down the hall and realized he had a full construction crew ready

>> WHAT THE HECK HAPPENED?

How did kids become so fat?

From food and technology, basically—more highly processed, sugary foods and drinks, less physical activity, and more reasons to sit on a couch, according to every expert we spoke to for this story.

Physical education can't cancel this out, but it can absolutely help. It's not just getting kids moving—the education part is equally important. "The goal of physical education is to educate people to the point at which, when given the choice, they'll voluntarily choose to be physically active," says George Graham, PhD, a past president of the National Association for Sport and Physical Education.

Okay, but what happened to phys ed? And why do so few kids take it?

"In the 1950s and '60s, physical education was respected as a way of life, whereas now it's part of aesthetic appeal," says Brian Grasso, president of the International Youth Conditioning Association. "Back then, phys-ed instructors were idealized in a hierarchy above lawyers and doctors, as they still are in the purest sport countries, such as Australia." Here, he says, the best fitness experts choose more profitable professions, such as working with collegiate and professional athletes.

Real trouble began in the 1970s. "Many adults had awful experiences with physical activity as kids, and now 'exercise' is a bad word to them," says Graham. The average American is not active and did not enjoy gym class. When phys ed failed the majority of American adults, he says, society as a whole began to conclude that it wasn't worthwhile.

Then we allowed legislatures to bury it. In the mid-'90s, states began academic testing, which pressured schools to cut "dispensable" programs. The No Child Left Behind Act of 2001, which tied funding to test scores, put more economic pressure on districts to focus on academics—often at the expense of physical education. "Ultimately," says Graham, "schools got the message: If it's not tested, it doesn't count."

to build platforms for weight-room equipment: Arrowhead's tech-ed department pitched in and saved the school more than $16,000.

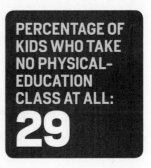

PERCENTAGE OF KIDS WHO TAKE NO PHYSICAL-EDUCATION CLASS AT ALL: 29

Contact your local private gym or college to see if the head trainer can help design a course or lead a weekly class. And reach out to local businesses to involve the community.

FACT: Experts are nearby.

PRESCRIPTION: Recruit them. Students will listen.

TURN THE GYM INTO A HEALTH CLUB

Club Arrowhead began as a summer-school program, and by the second year, "there were parents lined up at 4 a.m. with sleeping bags and lawn chairs for a 7 a.m. registration," says Steinbach.

The course consists of strength training, speed work, plyometrics, and flexibility. Coaches put the education back in physical education, explaining every facet, from the muscles used in an exercise to the point of dynamic warmups. Kids soak it up and exercise with a sense of purpose, not as though it's punishment.

Its popularity led to Club Arrowhead Fitness for Life, a cardiovascular course, and Adventure Phys Ed, a summer class that takes advantage of local resources—it includes backpacking, climbing, and canoeing in Wisconsin's lake country.

"We ought to be introducing kids to all kinds of different sports and activities," says George Graham, PhD, a past president of the National Association for Sport and Physical Education. Arrowhead's staff encourages students to suggest courses or activities. The faculty has received hundreds of suggestions, from rock climbing and bowling to table tennis.

You don't need a health-club budget to offer cool classes. The most successful schools are the ones that actively seek grants. Go to www. aahperd.org/naspe to learn more about this option.

FACT: Kids like variety.

PRESCRIPTION: Meet with administrators, teachers, and students to organize a fitness club at your high school.

OUTSOURCE AT LEAST ONE CLASS

As the physical-education system neared rock bottom in the late '90s, private fitness centers catering to kids charged onto the scene. Most were developed for young athletes, but parents began enrolling out-of-shape kids. By 2000, this niche market was a $4 billion business, roughly a quarter of the entire fitness industry in the United States, according to Brian Grasso, executive director of the International Youth Conditioning Association.

Loren Seagrave founded the first Velocity Sports Performance gym

▶▶HOW EXERCISE MAKES YOUR CHILD SMARTER

The fitter children are, the better their brains work. That's hard science from researchers at the University of Illinois at Urbana-Champaign, who tested elementary-school students.

Physically fit kids had greater P3 amplitude, a measurement of brain activity related to memory and focus, and faster P3 latency, meaning they were able to process information faster. "Parts of your brain don't develop until the late teenage years," says Charles H. Hillman, PhD, the study's lead author. "These data show that those who are fit are better able to use what they have."

Elementary-school students may have the most to gain from physical education. In a review of 44 studies examining the relationship between physical activity and cognition in children of varying ages, researchers at Arizona State University found that the youngest kids (grades one through five) improved cognitive development the most, followed by middle-school students.

The California Department of Education found that the fittest students in the state scored best on academic tests. For instance, the average reading score of students who achieved one of six goals on the statewide fitness evaluation was 38; students who achieved all six fitness goals averaged a reading score of 52.

At Arrowhead High School in Hartland, Wisconsin, organized exercise helped Corey Wise organize his schoolwork. "I started taking as much time with my homework as I did with my workout," he says. Class became fun, and it showed in his grades. Your child may benefit from planned activity, too.

in 1999. Now, with 77 facilities across North America and 20 more scheduled to open this year, the franchise is booming, and Seagrave is showcasing his training to schools. "Learning to accelerate, change direction, and jump higher is really exciting," he says. "When kids feel in control of their bodies, it gives them confidence."

Students at Hinsdale South High School, in Darien, Illinois, are bused to the local Velocity for a workout. Go to www.velocitysp.com to find a location near you. And visit the Internet sites of other national youth-fitness centers, such as Catz Training Centers (www.catzsports.com).

FACT: The private sector can help.

PRESCRIPTION: Survey your schools, gauge demand, and let free enterprise take over.

CALL A PARENT-TEACHER CONFERENCE

No longer assume a child is getting the physical education he or she needs. If you're a parent, approach your child's school principal to see how you can help; if you're faculty, involve the parents. "When my daughter told me in kindergarten that she ran 40 yards in a 30-minute class, I was pissed," says Liston. So he designed basic workout routines that any teacher or parent can lead. Go to www.menshealth.com/kids/ for a sample routine for elementary-school students.

Liston also held a silent auction to raise money for fitness equipment and to hire two part-time physical-education instructors for kindergarten through fifth grade. And he started Catz P.L.A.Y. (parents leading active youth), a program in which an active parent leads a physical-education class every Friday afternoon. Try these ideas at your school.

FACT: Schools won't change without a push from parents.

PRESCRIPTION: Get involved.

LOSE 10 POUNDS

Akins High School in Austin is straight out of *Stand And Deliver*. It's an impoverished Texas school where neither parents nor kids care enough about their health, says John Vogt, MS, CSCS, the physical-education instructor at the school. In his best Edward James Olmos impression, Vogt is piloting a Velocity-inspired course this fall.

"The objective is to generate interest and make examples of kids who excel," Vogt says. That can start at home. Vogt has a message for overweight coaches and parents: Get in shape. Vogt, 57, works out 3 or 4 days a week and encourages his staff to do the same.

FACT: Your example counts.

PRESCRIPTION: Drop a few.

≫THREE WAYS TO HELP YOUR KIDS EAT BETTER

Promise Academy, a charter school in Harlem, New York, closed its doors to vending machines and food brought in from outside. It serves only healthful food. Until your school does the same, it's up to you to take control. Use these simple strategies to help your kids eat healthfully.

Enroll in cooking class: And involve the kids. Children who learn about cooking learn about food. "Cooking classes open your mind to a variety of different ways to prepare healthy food," says Andrew Benson, head chef at Promise Academy. Benson offers a cooking class for parents and students; the children aren't the only ones who develop healthy habits. "Parents become interested in learning how to change their diets and their lives," he says. Go to www.cookingschools.com to find a class near you.

Make friends with a farmer: "If you go to a farmers' market, they'll usually give advice on how to prepare the foods," says Benson. Fresher food is more nutritious. And the closer a child is to the source of food, the more interested he or she will be in nutrition. That's crucial—because even children who consume excess calories have nutrient deficiencies. Canadian researchers found that 87 percent of kids don't get enough vitamin E, 28 percent lack magnesium, and 45 percent miss out on vitamin D. And a study in *Pediatrics* found that more than 60 percent of kids are calcium deficient, which, along with a lack of exercise, may have caused a rise in bone fractures.

Stop drinking soda: Stock up on milk and bottled water (if your tap water doesn't taste good). Kids get more than 50 percent of their beverages at home. When researchers at Children's Hospital Boston sent bottled water to families to replace their sugary drinks, kids lost about a pound a month. And a study in *Pediatrics* found that overweight preschool children are twice as likely to remain overweight if they drink sugar-sweetened beverages. Note that 100 percent juice is okay—it supplies fiber and key nutrients.

MY SUMMER OF STRENGTH

DISCOVER HOW A LONG-HAIRED HEADBANGER TAUGHT
MY BLOB OF FLABBY ADOLESCENCE TO LIGHTEN UP

BY COLIN McENROE

My son Joey has the kind of build that makes the high-school football coaches drool. As a sophomore, he tops 6 feet, with broad shoulders, a big chest, and thick wrists. I always notice those wrists, because I struggled through years of sports with wrists uncannily resembling Emily Dickinson's.

The coach made his first overture to Joey in eighth grade and quickly realized he was dealing with somebody who had absolutely no interest in spending the autumns of his youth getting his shins kicked by psychotic thugs who actually cared about the outcome of football games.

The coach gave up, and gradually I did, too. Joey played youth basketball for about five seasons and hated every one. On game days, his stomach flipped and flopped like a Slinky descending the Eiffel Tower.

So what? Not everybody is made for sports.

But there was another problem. Joey has a metabolism typical of Latino males (which he is). Nutritionists call it the "thrifty gene," adapted from ancient conditions of scarcity. His body stores calories, whereas mine might burn them. Eating a typical American diet and not doing much exercise, he's going to get fat. Which he did.

Everybody said he'd grow out of it at puberty. Instead, he grew taller but not thinner. He stopped swimming because he'd have to take off his shirt. One bittersweet night, he went swimming with me in the pool at my apartment complex, and I realized it was only because it was 10 p.m. and dark and no one was looking.

My ex-wife and I tried to control Joey's diet and coax him to exercise. This mainly involved getting him to do stuff with me at precisely the time in life when nobody wants to be seen with his dorky dad. Joey faces—in addition to my basic nerditude—the additional embarrassment of my being a white guy. Not all of his friends even know he has a white dad. When we're spotted together, he escapes shame by telling them I'm his probation officer.

So we would have a lot of conversations like this one:

Me: Wanna play tennis?

Him: No!

Me: C'mon!

Him: Where would we do it?

Me: The courts at your school.

Him: No way.

So, after long negotiation, we'd wind up at courts many miles away. I, of course, started to feel a little bit like somebody's mistress—the kind of date you can take only to restaurants in Brooklyn, where nobody knows either of you.

Food was the other problem. With no system in place, I would try to limit what he ate, which basically turned every strand of spaghetti into a bone of contention. And when you know somebody doesn't want you to eat, you tend to eat more, just in case you don't get another good chance.

As summer neared, we argued about how he would spend it. My plan involved camp counseling, summer school, and lots of exercise. His plan involved listening to suicide-exalting thrash music while IMing his friends on his computer and watching R-rated movies on HBO.

I sat down with him one day and said, "Let's put everything else on hold. And let's make this summer the time when you lose the weight. Let's do whatever it takes, and you'll go back in the fall looking like a new person."

Even in a lump of matter as inert as an American teenager, you can detect seismic shifts. He rearranged himself to accommodate a startling new idea.

"How is that possible?" he asked.

"I'll change my schedule around. We'll work out every day. We'll put you on a real diet. I'll get you a dietitian and trainer."

"And I'll look different?" The tone of hope that was stealing into his voice was heartbreaking. It made me realize how completely marooned he had been feeling.

"Yes. But only if we set up some rules and stick to them. The first one is that you have to stop gaming me and lawyering me. Every day, I will decide what we're going to do and where we're going to do it, and you'll go along with me, whether it strikes your fancy or not. The same goes for food. No arguing; no negotiating for bigger portions and better stuff. There won't be energy to waste on that."

He didn't even ask for time to think it over.

"Okay."

"Also, there's one person who could really help us," I said, echoing the tone of Ellen Burstyn when she decides to call in Max von Sydow to exorcise the demons from her child.

"Who is that?"

"You'll see."

Marlaine Philpotts is a registered dietitian, bodybuilder, co-owner of a weight-loss company called Diminishing Dimensions, blonde sports-car-driving babe and, in a pleasantly dominatrixy way, a scary person. There's something she does when you're not putting out—a kind of eerie coldness—that's much more intimidating than somebody yelling at you. Philpotts's company offers an exercise program for kids, and it's one of the few I've seen that's really serious. In a nation struggling with childhood obesity, there's a startling lack of good weight-loss programs for kids.

So I dragged Joey to meet Philpotts at a gym on Sunday and departed shortly thereafter so he wouldn't be able to triangulate with us. When I returned, Philpotts looked a little bit like von Sydow when he pops out of Linda Blair's bedroom, slumping against the wall and popping digitalis for his weak heart.

"I don't know if I can do this. I've never seen such negativity," she said.

"Give me an example."

"I told him he could shorten his life by being overweight, and he told me he has no interest in living past 30," she said, almost shaken.

"Pay no heed to that. He's just blustering because he's scared."

"Hmmm."

After consulting with both Philpotts and an endocrinologist, my ex-wife and I formulated a diet that completely eliminated sugar and almost all white flour, drastically cut carbs, increased fiber, and encouraged five small meals a day.

I quickly turned into something of a maniac about nutrition. I would troll the supermarket aisles, squinting at labels, comparing the sugar and carb counts in, say, various types of low-carb pasta. Around me would swirl an endless procession of wide Americans with elephantine butts, and in their carts would be a jumble of products in gaily colored packages, containing fats and sugars that they could not possibly consume without expanding to an even more terrifying size. I had to fight the urge to pull them over like a traffic cop and write them a ticket for speeding toward obesity: "Ma'am, do you know how fast you're going toward type-2 diabetes?"

I was right about Joey. When he went back to see Philpotts a week later, he had lost 3½ pounds. He was working out and following the diet.

She stared at him in puzzlement: "What happened? I thought you were going to be my worst client ever, but you take it more seriously than anybody else."

We split up the work. Philpotts taught him how to lift weights every Sunday afternoon. I took over the daily cardio. I kept it simple. Every weekday, we walked 5 miles, the same route at a local reservoir. In the afternoons, he'd lift. I quit my power yoga workouts, got up early, and worked from about 6 to 9 a.m. so I could take time off for a 9:30 walk. The 5 miles fell into a pattern of conversation: 1 mile of bitter arguing about my bossiness and his crummy attitude, 1 mile of arguing about who was more responsible for the bad feelings and disputatious nature of the day, 1 mile of dead silence for me while he listened to demonic screaming on his iPod, and then 2 miles of intensely important conversation.

And so it came to pass that what began as a quest to lose weight became a possibly more important summer of conversation between a father and a son verging on manhood. We talked religion, sex, politics, culture.

By summer's end, we had seen real progress. There were girls—pretty girls—in Joey's life. Not girlfriends, but girls who showed up and sat on the steps in front of his house and talked to him. This was a first. And when the endocrinologist weighed him at his next appointment, he had lost 20 pounds! The doctor was pleased but said he needed to lose 10 more by the following spring. And maybe 10 more after that.

PERCENTAGE OF MEN WHO SAY HOMER SIMPSON IS THE IDEAL TV DAD: 3

But as school got into gear, the morning walks slipped away. We argued about what to do, and I pushed him to find opportunities for exercise that did not depend on me. Some of the lost weight came back. He and Philpotts drifted apart. His shoulders hunched and his attitude darkened.

Joey had stopped believing in change and had, in particular, stopped believing that my ideas were any good. I was a guy who did yoga, was in love with a woman, listened to John Mayer. He was a guy who did nothing, loved nobody, and listened to music that made Slipknot sound like Air Supply. What could a creature of the dark learn from me, a person of the light? With my hobbitlike hairy feet and sunny outlook, I was, nonetheless, the dad of an Orc.

What could I do?

Across the street from where I work, a new health club emerged, a Malibu Fitness joint. At first, I ruled out taking Joey there because it looked bright and sunny and happy, the kind of place he would hate.

And then I got desperate. I booked him an hour with a personal trainer.

He blew up at me. How could I do that without consulting him?

"If I had asked you, you would have said no," I told him. "Look, you win. This is the last time I will force exercise on you. From now on, if you want a workout, you'll have to ask for it. But I paid for this one, so you're going."

"Good," he snarled. "That means I'm all done with this stuff forever."

I dropped him off the next afternoon. His eyes darted suspiciously around the happy, white, Richard Meier–style building—his idea of hell. His trainer, somebody named Ryan Oliver, hadn't arrived yet. The staff had him warm up on a Lifecycle, and I ducked out before he could pick another fight with me.

He stumbled into my office about 90 minutes later.

"You won't believe this," he said, "but I really want to go back. I want to go twice a week. It has to be that guy, though. Ryan. Nobody else."

I went back the next day and signed him up. And I met Ryan.

Not a big guy. About 20. Slicked-back hair. Narrow eyes. Vampire tattoo on his neck. If you and he were the only ones on a subway platform at night, you'd be nervous. The gym owner told me he's into an extreme martial art called ground fighting. I looked it up. Eeww! It's about as far from yoga as you can get.

"You got through to my kid in a way that nobody else has," I told Ryan.

"We like a lot of the same music," he said with an evil smile. You have no idea what a scary statement that is. We're talking about guys in goalie masks cutting up frozen buffalo with chain saws. And that's the string section.

Joey had found a fellow Orc.

"He's actually a very nice young man," the owner assured me later. "He teaches Spinning, too."

I didn't care if he was nice or not. I wrote a big fat check for 11 more sessions. And now they are training together; they may be training to overthrow society for all I know. Fine. I had stumbled onto the answer. Since my positive messages were getting nowhere, I had to meet his darkness with more darkness.

"You can use the gym, too," the owner said. "Who knows? Your son might want you to come and work out with him sometime."

"He won't," I said. "Unless he gets stronger than me. Then he'll want me to come over so he can show me up."

"Oh," said the owner, "I've seen your son. He will get stronger than you."

LOSE THE LUBE

Couples having difficulty conceiving may want to pitch the KY. New research from the Cleveland Clinic shows that several popular lubricants can significantly decrease the motility of sperm and possibly damage their DNA. In lab tests, Replens, Astroglide, FemGlide, and KY Jelly were the worst offenders. Your best bet: Pre-Seed, which caused no significant problems in the study.

CALL U-HAUL NOW

You don't have to be hit by a bus to be killed by one. British researchers studied the medical records of 22,500 children and learned that those living near bus or train stations had 12 times the cancer risk of other kids. Diesel-engine fumes may be to blame.

STOP THE SPERM

Scientists have made two baby steps—oops—toward reversible male contraception. First, men who received contraceptive hormonal injections had an 83 percent chance of recovering their normal sperm counts after 1 year, the *Lancet* reported. The androgen injections suppress sperm production. Availability is at least 5 years away.

Then there's the Intra Vas Device (IVD), which plugs each vas deferens, the tube that carries sperm from the testicles. The device has worked in animals, and the government has approved human tests. "It's basically a kinder, gentler vasectomy" with potentially better reversibility, says Elaine Lissner, of the Male Contraception Information Project. Availability is several years away.

MAKE ROOM FOR TWO

The older your wife is when she gets pregnant, the greater the chance that she'll give birth to fraternal twins, say researchers at the Free University Medical Center, in the Netherlands. Their study of 507 women found that women older than 30 are more likely than younger women to have twins, because their bodies produce more follicle-stimulating hormone. Levels of this hormone increase with age to help ovaries release eggs, sometimes leading to double ovulation.

START 'EM YOUNG

Being physically active makes kids smarter and more confident, according to a report in the journal *Pediatrics*. A study of 11,957 teenagers found that those who played sports were less likely to participate in risky behaviors or have low self-esteem.

Athletic kids also had better grades, report the researchers at the University of Minnesota and University of North Carolina. The most likely reason: Teens who are active are exposed to team building and can see the benefits of hard work.

"Instead of having family TV time, build in time when the family is active together," suggests study coauthor Penny Gordon-Larsen, PhD.

GET THE ALL CLEAR

Make sure to confirm that your vasectomy worked—but not by playing sperm roulette. A shocking 80 percent of men who have vasectomies don't go for their "all clear" semen tests 12 weeks later, new research shows. That's risky, because sperm can live in your plumbing for up to 3 months after the operation. The Cleveland Clinic reports that men are skipping one or both of the recommended doctor visits at 8 and 12 weeks. Researcher Stephen Jones, MD, says the 12-week test is critical.

PLAN AHEAD

Before you hit 40 is the best age to conceive, according to a new study by French researchers. Their study of nearly 2,000 couples undergoing fertility treatments suggests that men age 40 or older are 70 percent less likely to get their wives pregnant than men who are younger than 30, regardless of the woman's age. An age-related decline in sperm quantity and quality may be to blame, say researchers.

GO FOR A STROLLER

Some serious runners balk at jogging strollers. But a new study in the *Journal of Sports Medicine and Physical Fitness* found that running while pushing a stroller burns more calories and doesn't hurt your running form. Researchers had 10 athletes run with and without a stroller for 30 minutes. The added resistance of the stroller boosted both their heart rates and lactate concentrations without affecting stride length.

"Physiologically, no negatives come from pushing a stroller," says study author John Smith, PhD, who recommends a one-armed grip. "The opposite arm is then free to swing, helping to counterbalance your legs."

BE GLAD FOR HEIGHT

Princeton researchers have learned that tall people tend to be more intelligent than their shorter peers. After reviewing 30 years' worth of cognitive tests taken by children under age 3, they found that lankier kids earned higher scores on average. The same kids also chose more lucrative careers as adults. Scientists think nutrition in utero may be related to both smarts and height.

TRY TO GET ALONG

Fighting with your wife could hurt your kids' grades, suggests a new study from Auburn University College of Human Sciences. In the study of 54 couples, researchers recorded the frequency and intensity of marital conflicts and then monitored each couple's children through 7 nights of sleep. The result: Kids in families with moderate to severe mom–dad arguing lost an average of 30 minutes of sleep per night. Sleep loss can contribute to poor school performance and increased adjustment problems, says lead study author Mona El-Sheikh.

JUST RELAX

Setting rigid rules may lead to larger kids. A Boston University study of 872 children determined that authoritative adults were more likely to have overweight kids than were more permissive parents. A high-stress household can cause children to overeat, even if exercise and healthy eating are emphasized.

WHAT'S NEW

MOVIEBEAM

Until the high-def DVD format war plays out, we'll watch from our couches. This Disney-backed set-top box delivers future-proof high definition with a rotation of 100 classics and new releases, picked up for $2 to $5 each from existing TV towers. No contract, no commitment, no problem. ($250. www.moviebeam.com)

DUCANE 3-BURNER GRILL

This stainless-steel grill packs in 624 square inches of cooking space, a side burner, and a motorized rotisserie spit, for a pittance. ($720. www.ducane.com)

PARENTAL SURVEILLANCE DEVICE

There's nothing like being 17 and invincible. Remember the feeling? Cruising through town with the top down, radio blasting, three people squeezed in front and five more in the back, weaving in and out of traffic. Now stop and picture your teenager at the wheel. Scary? It should be. Automobile accidents are the leading cause of death among adolescents, claiming almost 6,000 teens in 2004 (the last year for which records are available)—more than double the number lost to the next leading cause of death, homicide. Now there's a way to surreptitiously monitor your kid's driving habits with the tiny new CarChip ($139 to $197). The size of a 9-volt battery, this gadget plugs into your car's onboard diagnostic port, used to capture information about the automobile's performance and found in all post-1996 cars.

The device records up to 300 hours of performance data (how fast and how far the car is going, fuel consumption, hard accelerations and decelerations). There's also an optional alarm feature, which can be set to go off when the driver exceeds a specific speed, acceleration, or braking limit. Kind of like an electronic version of . . . you.

PANASONIC LUMIX DMC-L1 CAMERA

The unrivaled color quality of a digital SLR comes at the expense of one of digital photography's key benefits: the ability to frame your shot on the LCD. That's because their massive light sensors suck up so much power that the screen can spring to life only after the shot is taken. This 7.5 megapixel digital solves that problem by adding a second light sensor that doesn't rob power from the first. ($349. www.panasonic.com)

SONY HDR-HC3 CAMCORDER

This high-resolution (1080i) camcorder minimizes the space crunch with a palm-size footprint and a 1-pound weight. It's the best bang for the bulk in high-definition video recording. ($1,500. www.sonystyle.com)

READY, SET, ACTION

FIVE WAYS TO MAKE HOME MOVIES WORTH WATCHING

1. **TELL A STORY:** "It gets boring without reason and story," says IMAX filmmaker Gordon Brown. When you edit, you need cutaway footage to build anticipation and add depth. Don't just film the climax—shoot bits of the backstory; interview the main players throughout the action; and show the reactions of bystanders.

2. **OVERSHOOT:** "It makes for interesting filmmaking when you're running off of instinct; you don't have time to intellectualize shots, so you just do them," says Stacy Peralta, director of *Dogtown and Z-Boys*. Your ratio of footage to edited tape should be at least 2 to 1. "Don't be afraid to overshoot; this gives you the freedom to figure out what will work best with the action."

3. **MATCH MUSIC:** "Music sets your film's emotional tenor," says Peralta. "It tells people what they should feel." Pick your music first and edit around it; it's far easier than trying to slap a song on already cut footage. "If you play music against type and play calm music during frenzied action, the results can be amazing," says Dave Knox, Hollywood cinematographer.

4. **KEEP MOVING:** A static camera stagnates the action, so keep your rig in motion. "It puts the audience in the scene," says Peralta. If you're filming on a street, carry the camera on a skateboard or bicycle, or hold it out the window of a car. If you're at an amusement

park, film your kids from the carriage of a Ferris wheel. Zooming is not motion—it screams "amateur."

5. **STAY AHEAD OF THE ACTION:** "Lead" the frame by placing the subject on one side and leaving wide open space on the side to which he's moving.

⟫DIRECTOR LINGO

Sound like a pro with these director buzzwords.

Establishing shot: A long, wide-angle shot that introduces the setting.

Head-on shot: When the subject moves straight at the camera.

Kodak courage: The sense of invincibility that a camera instills.

Magic hour: The perfect half hour or so at sunset when everything is draped in an orange glow.

Put it on the sticks: Docking the camera on a tripod for a static shot.

Smash cut: A sudden, dramatic edit meant to surprise the viewer.

I fell asleep in the hot tub last night. Could I have cooked my sperm or even made the boys infertile?

Heating your scrotum could temporarily decrease the size of your swim team, says *Men's Health* urology advisor Larry I. Lipshultz, MD. Since it takes the testicles about 3 months to complete one cycle of sperm production, it'll take about that long for your count to return to normal. But return it will.

What's the best timing to ensure my wife gets pregnant?

Every woman's cycle is slightly different, but generally, a woman has the greatest chance of becoming pregnant anywhere between the 8th and 16th days of her cycle. Since you're trying for a baby, have sex no more than every other day.

"If a couple has very frequent sex, there's not enough time for sperm to build up in the ejaculate," says Paula Castaño, MD, an assistant clinical professor of obstetrics and gynecology at Columbia University. "He may be, in essence, shooting blanks." If the math is too confusing, buy an ovulation predictor kit. They're sold at most drugstores and are similar to the urine tests used to detect pregnancy.

Do at-home fertility tests work?

Yes and no, says Dr. Lipshultz. Women can monitor ovulation with a urine test, and a semen test will tell you if your sperm count hits 20 million per milliliter. But neither test can pinpoint a problem. Men should see a urologist for tests to determine their levels of the hormones that control sperm production.

Are there any toys or games that can make my toddler daughter smarter?

Toy manufacturers such as Baby Einstein and LeapFrog would have you believe so, but their products are no better than the boxes they come in when it comes to building a child's brain.

"What makes toddlers smarter isn't the toy itself; it's the rich stimulation they receive from other people, particularly caregivers," says Susan Landry, PhD, chief of developmental pediatrics at the University of Texas Health Science Center at Houston. A recent follow-up study of 1,795 3-year-olds found that those who explored their environment, engaged with other children, and verbally interacted with adults scored 12 points higher on total IQ at age 11 than did their less curious and less social peers.

When your child picks up a new toy, sit down with her and make it a multilevel learning experience. If it's a pop-up toy, for example, say, "What happens when you turn the red knob? The weasel pops up! What sound does the weasel make?" Right there you've introduced the color red, cause and effect, and sound association. "The more information you give her, the more she'll absorb, particularly if it's through verbal interaction with you," says Landry. And if your kid happens to prefer the ribbon from the gift wrapping to the present itself, let her play with it (but make sure she doesn't choke herself with it). Nurturing her creative streak will do more good than having her master the latest gadget.

My wife and I are having a son. I want him circumcised. She doesn't. Is one way better than the other, health-wise?

PERCENTAGE OF MEN WHO SAY FRED FLINTSTONE IS THE IDEAL TV DAD:

4

No. Some physicians might tell you that circumcision can prevent urinary-tract infections in infants and reduce the risk of penile cancer and STD transmission in adults, but the situation isn't that clear-cut, so to speak.

"After looking at 40 years of research, we

found that the health benefits are not so significant as to create a national recommendation to circumcise," says Alan Fleischman, MD, a member of the American Academy of Pediatrics' task force on circumcision.

However, recent research by Yale researchers found a new reason to forgo the foreskin: They determined that adult men who are circumcised are less likely than uncircumcised men to contract HIV from an infected partner. The foreskin contains cell receptors that act as targets for the virus to latch onto, which is why transmission rates are higher among men who missed the cut.

Of much greater concern are the procedure's sexual repercussions. When a doctor performs a circumcision, "he removes up to 50 percent of the skin on the penile shaft—skin that would normally grow into about 12 square inches of highly erogenous tissue," says Ronald Goldman, PhD, executive director of the Circumcision Resource Center (www.circumcision.org) in Boston. "Men circumcised as adults describe the difference in pleasure as seeing in black-and-white as opposed to color." Studies also show, says Goldman, that the experience can have long-term psychological repercussions, ranging from sexual phobias to post-traumatic stress disorder.

That said, if you yourself are circumcised or support the procedure on religious grounds, you might still want to lobby your wife in favor of circumcision. "Boys who grow up cut differently than their fathers or community members can be affected emotionally and psychologically," says Dr. Fleischman. "That needs to be taken into account when the final choice is made."

Someone killed the Santa myth for my kid. How can I restore it?

Don't bother. "If you go out of the way to perpetuate the myth, it will confuse the child's ability to believe you about more important matters," says Daniel Amen, MD, a *Men's Health* mental-health advisor. "Lying about Santa makes it okay to lie about other things, as well."

To ease the blow, listen actively. Ask little Johnny where he heard that St. Nick is a fraud. Ask what he thinks. If he still wants to believe, don't explode the myth, Dr. Amen says. "He might want to be in denial." So talk around it, leaving him some mental wiggle room.

Dr. Amen's script: "There are many wonderful traditions that we celebrate, and we're not sure if they are all true, because we weren't there when they started." And talk about other things that make the holidays magical. Like giving—talk about how it helps people connect to others and feel special, Dr. Amen suggests. But really, don't lie. "It just sets them up to mistrust you later on," he says. Kids are pretty smart. They'll figure it out eventually, with you or without you.

How do I tell my kids the family dog died?

There's nothing sadder than losing a beloved family dog—except for having to break the news to your kids. Often the children's first brush with death, the passing of a pet provides an opportunity to shape how they'll handle life's bigger tragedies. Start with honesty. "They're going to find out the truth anyway," says Wallace Sife, a psychologist and the head of the Association for Pet Loss and Bereavement (www.aplb.org). "In many cases," says Dr. Sife, "your children will remember [a lie] with great resentment, anger, or pain."

Hold a family meeting to decide on a memorial. This gathering is also an ideal time to talk about where a chiweenie's soul goes. Stress the notion that all of you are better for having known Fido. Make sure you grieve yourself. If you don't, you may belittle your children's feelings. (Remember, your kids look to you for cues on how to act.) Don't rush into replacing the family pooch. When you do get a new dog, include your kids in the decision. After all, they've been through a lot.

I have a beautiful wife, two wonderful kids, and a great house—and yet I feel utterly trapped. Sometimes I want out. Why?

The problem might not be your wife or your kids or your house or even you. The problem might be your job. "Each year, men take on 10 percent more responsibilities in every aspect of their lives than they had the year before," says Jim Conway, PhD, author of *Men in Crisis* and founder of Midlife Dimensions, a counseling service in Fullerton, California. It's part of the natural process of maturing. But by the time they reach their mid-forties, the cumulative stress of those responsibilities can be overwhelming, particularly when it comes to their jobs, which often become the tipping point upon which a peaceful midlife transition tumbles into a full-blown midlife crisis.

"About 75 percent of a man's identity is wrapped up in his career," explains Dr. Conway. "But he can't blame his work for his unhappiness— that would be like blaming himself. Instead, he shifts the blame to his family and says, 'I want out.'" And that inevitably leads to the cliché of the 50-year-old guy on the bar stool, flipping through a tattered family album and wondering where it all went wrong.

Don't let that be you. The difference between a job and a family is that a job can't love you back. Unless there are serious and irreconcilable problems at home, that's where you need to put your energies. If that notion conflicts with your job, consider changing careers (frightening, yes, but most people do it at least once) or sliding sideways into another opportunity. "I often see guys go into consulting or become entrepreneurs and finally start that business they've always dreamed of," says Dr. Conway. But don't spend too much time focusing on yourself: New research from Cornell University suggests that middle-aged women are even more likely than men to go through "turbulent midlife transitions."

Bullies keep picking on my kid. Should I get him boxing lessons?

No. A study of 500 preteen boys in Norway found that those who took up boxing were five times more likely to fight, steal, and skip school than kids in less combative sports. But that doesn't mean you should tell your kid to turn the other cheek. "Get him martial-arts lessons," says Larry Koenig, PhD, author of *Smart Discipline: Fast, Lasting Solutions for Your Child's Self-Esteem and Your Peace of Mind.*

The true power behind martial arts like karate and kung fu comes

PERCENTAGE OF KIDS WHO ARE OVERWEIGHT OR OBESE:

45

not from a roundhouse kick to the solar plexus (however handy) but rather from their philosophies of non-aggression. "They teach respect," says Dr. Koenig. "Research shows that, in so doing, martial arts improve a child's self-esteem and the way he carries himself— two weaknesses a bully homes in on when selecting a target." In fact, a Florida Atlantic University study of 189 children ages 7 to 13 found that those with high self-confidence were less likely to be picked on than their less-confident peers.

If your child does get picked on, address the issue with him immediately, even if it's just teasing. "Parents often tell their kids that it's no big deal, that it's just kids being kids," says Dr. Koenig. "Nothing can be further from the truth. Words can be far more difficult to get over than a black eye." Researchers at the Oregon Research Institute agree. In a study of 223 kids, they found that verbally harassed middle schoolers were three times more likely to abuse alcohol in high school.

Here's the best way to deal with teasing: Tell your child to just agree with it. If, for example, a bully calls your kid a sissy, tell him to respond, "Yeah, I am." Next to self-confidence, agreeableness is the most powerful antibully tool. "If you're not pushing back, they have nothing to fight against," says Dr. Koenig.

Any tips for a dad who is working away from home half the time?

Yes, find another job. Don't underestimate how important you are to your family. Kids grow up fast, and you owe it to them to be present, especially in their formative years. Until you can find a solution that keeps you at home more often, consider these ideas:

Let the kids know where you are going. Download Google Earth. You can zoom in on the roof of the hotel where you'll be staying. The kids can print it and show off to their friends. It gives them a sense of control and connection to you.

Leave a gift or note for each child to find when you're away.

Buy them cell phones to help you stay in touch. Try to talk to them before school and bedtime every day. E-mail is another way to stay connected. Say "I love you" often to reassure them of their importance to you. When you get home, be completely present for each member of your family, especially your wife.

Are video games ruining my son's brain?

Just make sure his life isn't all carjacking and hookers. James Gee, PhD, a professor of education at the University of Wisconsin and the author of *What Video Games Have to Teach Us about Learning and Literacy*, says, "If the child is playing sports, reading books, and playing video games—and especially if he is relating with other kids—then that's fine." Multiplayer games like Civilization or Halo can teach business and organizational skills. The Sims can fire the imagination, and a game like Age of Mythology can spark an interest in the subject.

How concerned should I be that my kids will get caught illegally swapping music files online?

From a statistical standpoint, not very. The Recording Industry Association of America has sued about 15,000 illegal file-sharers since September 2003, a drop in the bucket compared with the estimated 6 million Americans on peer-to-peer (P2P) networks such as LimeWire or Kazaa at any time. Also, the RIAA doesn't target downloaders but rather uploaders. (Note: On most P2P sites, you download and upload simultaneously.) The odds are good, though, that your kids will get caught by spyware or viruses, which can slow or even take over your computer. Bottom line: Encourage your kids to pay for music through services like iTunes (www.itunes.com) or unlimited-download sites like Yahoo! Music (www.music.yahoo.com).

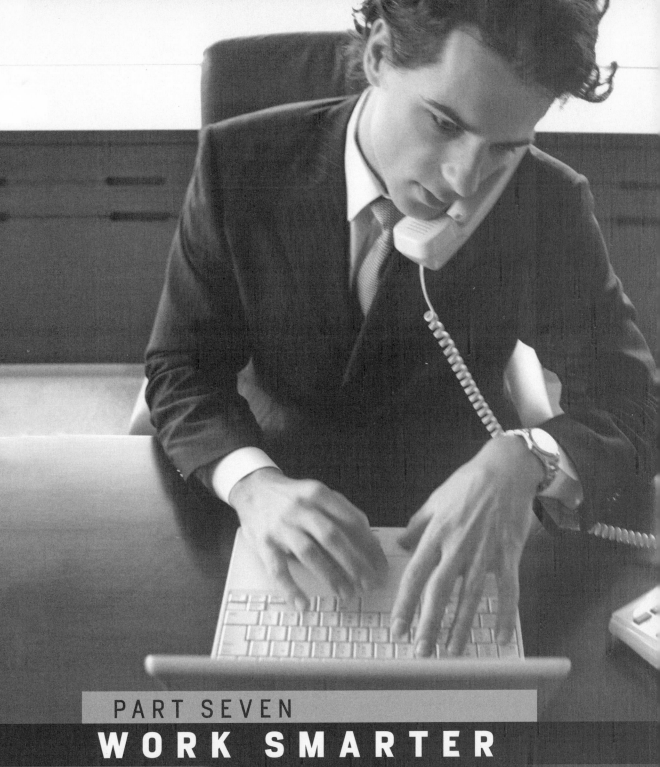

PART SEVEN

WORK SMARTER

THE PROMOTION PLAN

FOLLOW THESE SEVEN STEPS TO A BIGGER SALARY

BY GIL SCHWARTZ

A few years ago, I was a director-level 'droid slaving away for the kind of bucks some people pay as the luxury tax on their BMWs.

I would attend management meetings—since I was part of that group in everything but title, salary, and perks—and all would go well until the last couple of hours, when I'd be called upon to leave the room so the big boys could talk about options and bonuses. It really steamed my latte. I was determined to join their club.

So I did what I thought I should do: I asked. It's not a bad beginning, as we'll discuss in a moment. "Gee," said my boss, "you're a worthy candidate to be a vice president, but guess what? We're not making them anymore. Human Resources said so."

"What?" I asked. "You lost the mold or something?"

"No," said my boss. "But it's late in the year, and the swallows are headed off to Capistrano Beach, and blah blah blah," and I stopped listening because I saw I was headed nowhere.

This went on for months. Then it just so happened I was called upon to do some kind of industry symposium where people who have a couple of ideas about something address a bunch of folks who have no

PERCENTAGE OF MEN WHO SAY RESPECT AT WORK IS MORE IMPORTANT THAN MONEY OR POWER:

82

ideas about anything. After the session, people came around and showed me their teeth and patted my back and said I'd done okay. My boss saw that. A week later, I was named vice president. Today, I stand atop my function, with no particular place to go from here. But that's another story.

Careers are like sharks. They either move forward—eating, growing, becoming ever more dangerous and toothy—or fall to the bottom of the professional ocean and die, to be eaten by other, more viable careers in that great circle of work life. So getting a promotion is not, as it may seem at first blush, an issue of simply improving what you have. It's a matter of survival.

Here, then, is a simple path to promotion that is guaranteed—unless, of course, you're a total gomer.

STEP 1: MAKE GREAT NOISE

It's amazing how many people languish in their current positions because they go straight to seething. A worthwhile employee who asks the boss for a step up is almost never resented. In fact, the request makes the fearful delegator you work for imagine for one horrible moment what life would be like without you. I can tell you this: I'm a squeaky wheel, and I've found that just about every time I've squeaked, I've eventually been greased.

Of course, you must have some purchase on reality.

A few years ago, I worked with a woman who was truly terrible. I'll call her Betty. Betty arrived at the office each morning with huge bags under her eyes and an invisible noose around her neck. During the day, she talked on the phone with her mother, her shrink, her equally disgruntled pals across corporate America. Her work was spotty, off-the-wall, and at times nonexistent.

The day came when we were effecting one of those head-count reductions that always happen around Christmas, and when we looked at the org chart, there was one gaping, steaming crater in it named Betty. "Will you miss her?" my boss asked the table of executioners, who were sharing a Danish spread. No one said yes.

So, on the day we were announcing the reductions, Betty asked to see me. She knows, I thought to myself, and felt a little relieved. It's nice when people know. It saves you so much pain. I called her in.

"I've been here for nearly 2 years," Betty began, "and I think it's about time I got a promotion." I know it's insensitive, but I almost burst out laughing. Betty was living proof that some people truly don't have a clue. Don't be one of those people.

STEP 2:
TAKE A PILE OF CRAP OFF YOUR BOSS'S PLATE

Many losers believe they deserve a promotion simply because they've been around long enough and management should be loyal to them. Ha! Management, loyal? It's all about production, consistency, and drive, guys.

The quality of work that gets you promoted is the kind that makes it unnecessary for your boss to do anything but manage. Let me give you an example. Four times a year, my pal Morrison's boss had to write up what the finance division had done during the previous quarter. It required applying English sentences to financial spreadsheets, and it was a truly terrible task for a guy like Morrison's boss, a deal-making b.s. artist who rose to the top by crunching numbers like baby ants. As soon as Morrison achieved manager-level grunt, he said to his boss, "Hey, if you don't mind, I'd like to take a stab at the narrative on the third quarter, okay?"

The boss's lower lip began trembling, and a rivulet of spittle ran down his chin, so deep was his shock and sudden rush of hope. "Yes, sure," he mumbled. The narrative came out fine—nothing brilliant, because it didn't really have to be. The fact that it was done at all, and that the vice president had 27½ more hours to look out the window and be vice presidential? That was all that mattered. My pal is a director now, with

AVERAGE NUMBER OF VACATION DAYS EACH AMERICAN RECEIVES PER YEAR:

12

his eye on his boss's chair. After all, the guy can't live forever. He can't even write a coherent paragraph!

STEP 3: TRADE UP YOUR MEETING SCHEDULE

If you gather with tiny toads, you're just another little green blob on the lily pad. Remember: Any functional senior officer has so many silly meetings, he feels like screaming by 3 p.m. every day. Look at his agenda and see what kind of neat stuff you can cherry-pick.

Naturally, you're not going to nab the big, showy stuff. His sit-down with the chairman about future new revenue streams is not one he'll fork over. But the gathering in the dead of winter, way across town? The one he agreed to attend without really thinking about it? Or the meeting with accounting or research or public relations about something he can't remember? Well, there will be at least six vice presidents at those things, and while that's not a glamorous prospect for your boss, it is for you. Suddenly, you're surrounded by your betters, and, if you manage these opportunities with distinction, who's to say that you shouldn't, before too long, be one of them?

STEP 4: WEAR RAW, NAKED AMBITION ON YOUR SLEEVE

Be a pain in the ass, damn it! For every 10 things you do to make your boss happy, prod him once. Keep in mind that nobody in the business world disrespects the man who is purely ambitious. I take that back. There is one kind, and he may be your boss, so tread lightly.

I used to work for a guy I'll call Barber. He was not a serious player. The business had changed a lot in the few years we'd worked together. I had changed with it. He hadn't. He was a big meeting junkie, pressing people for "deliverables" and other schweck that meant something in a prior generation of corporate America. Everybody knew his meetings were a waste of time, but you couldn't get out of them. What you could do was sleep through them or, more likely, send fellow meeting nerds to them while you, the true operating guy, went to lunch.

And so it was that Barber had his meetings that came to nothing, and the executives who didn't have time for that crap dealt with me. Pretty soon, I was the go-to guy. I made the right level of noise about getting another stripe, but Barber wasn't biting. After all,

MINIMUM NUMBER OF DAYS OF ANNUAL PAID LEAVE REQUIRED BY LAW IN THE EUROPEAN UNION:

28

stripes were all he had. So I languished until, as these things happen, there was another merger, another go-round in the great dance of acquisition and divestiture, and then all the guys who were looking for the genuine deal turned to me.

What I'm saying is this: No amount of asking is going to make a difference if your boss feels like your career advancement is not aligned with his self-interest. So you might want to be a little more careful than I was. Or not. In the end, what goes around comes home to roost.

STEP 5:
DRESS LIKE A HITTER

There's an old rule in the world of facades and mirrors we play in: You have to dress at least one level better than your true station would dictate. This can be expensive, but it's worth it. I'm going to take a second here to quote someone who is all too rarely cited in business conversation. The world would be a better place if people drew on Shakespeare with the same verve that they did Trump. Here's what perhaps the smartest man who ever worked a court had to say on the subject:

Costly thy habit as thy purse can buy,

But not expressed in fancy; rich, not gaudy;

For the apparel oft proclaims the man.

I'll translate: Spend as much as you can on your clothes. Don't be showy; just look good, because your clothes speak of who you are. Your clothes should say, in a low, persuasive, mature voice, "Wow. Look at Bob. He really should be a vice president," and even, "I wonder where he

PERCENTAGE DECREASE IN RISK OF DYING OF HEART DISEASE IF YOU GO ON VACATION AT LEAST ONCE A YEAR:

29

got that tie," or, in the case of New Media, "that T-shirt."

STEP 6:
GO OUT AND PLAY
(BUT WATCH OUT FOR TRAFFIC)

The world is a very big place. There are all kinds of people in it—people who may appreciate you even if others do not. This is not to say that you need to be shopping yourself all over creation. Looking for a job elsewhere is a risky way of seeking a promotion at your beloved place of employment, because if you actually float your dinghy into foreign waters, you have to be prepared to stay there.

I knew a very wormy guy once—let's call him Gary. He'd been at his marketing firm for a pretty long time and achieved a certain level of stature. After a while, he started thinking he deserved better. So he looked around, found an offer that he didn't really want to take at a firm without the cachet of his own, figured hey, what the heck, went to his boss, and said, "I've been offered a better title and money at a place down the street, and I wonder if you'd like to match it." And his boss stood up, offered his chubby paw, and said, "Nah, but good luck to you, Gary. You'll do great over there." So Gary had to go. He's freelancing now.

What you want is not a strategy built around threats and dueling

▶▶DELEGATION TRICK #457

For best results, delegate tasks instead of responsibilities. What's the difference? A task has a specific beginning and end, and its success or failure can be easily gauged. Example: "I need you to compile this month's Wanger report and have your draft to me by Friday." This is far better than "You're in charge of Wangers from now on." In the latter case, your subordinate's interest will inevitably wane—after all, it's not his reputation on the line—and your Wanger will no longer impress.

offers. What you want is to step into the real world and meet people, and be a player, and make sure you're treated as such. Eat in the right places, where people can see you and think, Gee, I didn't know Ned was a hitter. Have drinks in the little establishments where the powerful go to get sodden. Attend conferences and ask the organizers whether there are little panels you can sit on. You think the people who appear at those things are any smarter than you? They're not. They just (that's right) asked.

> **PERCENTAGE OF MEN WHO WANT TO STAY IN THEIR CURRENT JOB ONLY "UNTIL SOMETHING BETTER COMES ALONG":**
> **60**

It was, in the end, my profile in the "real world" that seduced management into promoting me to the land where options are not a dream and bonuses buy time-shares in remote locations. If I had been nothing but an inside guy, I never would have made it beyond the branches I could reach on tiptoe.

STEP 7:
BAIL

In the end, when all else fails, when you feel disrespected every day and guys with bad hair are making twice your coin, you may need to join another corporate nation. Find something you really and truly want, and then say goodbye. Who knows? The knowledge that they blew it, that you truly are not posturing or cutting an attitude but are genuinely out of there, may turn your bosses into slabs of malleable cheese, willing to do anything to convince you to stay. That's the kind of problem I hope you have one day.

Me, I'll just wave to you from where I am, perched pretty much where I guess you'd like to be. When you get here, I'll be glad to see you, I suppose. Though, to tell you the truth, you guys kind of scare me.

MENTOR MIRROR

WHICH LEADER ARE YOU? FIND YOUR MENTOR;
SEE YOUR FUTURE

BY GIL SCHWARTZ

Throughout human history, it's been the fate, honor, or curse of certain men to lead others to glory, success, or destruction—even if they weren't the smartest, fastest, or best equipped. In many ways, it's the pressure of responsibility that makes a man, raising some to greatness and turning others into the warped, gnarled weirdos who pass for executive officers down the hall from you. Which way will it break for you? Just figure out whose footsteps you're following.

THE ALL-STAR:
AUGUSTUS, FIRST ROMAN EMPEROR

Augustus surrounded himself with his enemies, gave them respect and power, and kept his eye on them until he could take them out. It takes patience, toughness, and vision to be Augustus, and these qualities don't come along often in one person. Are you that person?

PRIMARY BENEFIT: You know what's going on pretty much all the time.

BIGGEST DOWNSIDE: People tend to disappoint you.

HOW TO KNOW IF YOU'RE THIS LEADER: Junior guys follow you like baby ducks.

THE LUSTY TYRANT:
HENRY VIII, KING OF ENGLAND

The Catholic Church wouldn't grant Henry VIII a divorce, so Henry replaced it with a church of his own creation. He then went about persecuting Catholics, because he enjoyed crushing his enemies. He was so disappointed with a succession of wives that he chopped off the heads of a few of them. You could be a Henry—lustful, large, in charge, a man to fear and suck up to, one who shapes the world around him to suit his needs. It does, however, require you to be morbidly obese.

PRIMARY BENEFIT: You don't see problems, you see opportunities.

BIGGEST DOWNSIDE: You always have garlic breath.

HOW TO KNOW IF YOU'RE THIS LEADER: You order a nice big appetizer at every lunch, and you always see if the server is single.

THE BOY WONDER:
ALEXANDER, LEADER OF THE GREEKS

Alexander generously, if violently, spread the glory of Greece throughout the known world, even to people who were doing quite well without it. For him, leadership was the hunt, the kill, the flag flying above the ramparts. The world has a place for such people. They die young and leave beautiful corpses, but they have a good time while they reign. You could be one of them. You just have to want one thing bad enough: more.

PRIMARY BENEFIT: You have the world on a string at age 3.

BIGGEST DOWNSIDE: You hit the glass ceiling at 30.

HOW TO KNOW IF YOU'RE THIS LEADER: You can either make a deal or kill somebody on the elevator ride to the 40th floor.

THE VISIONARY REFORMER:
PETER THE GREAT, CZAR OF RUSSIA

His backward nation was bordered by the most affluent and educated entity the world had known to that point, so he opened his doors to Europe's best and brightest engineers, architects, and merchants. He was also no weenie. Convinced that Russia needed a port on the Baltic Sea, he started a war with Sweden, which he won 21 years later, and founded St. Petersburg. You could be like Peter—liberal, philosophical, open to new ideas, brutal if necessary. You could do worse.

PRIMARY BENEFIT: You feel great satisfaction at bringing your organization out of the dark ages.

BIGGEST DOWNSIDE: Lots of reactionary jerks try to rain on your parade.

HOW TO KNOW IF YOU'RE THIS LEADER: You see things that need to be done and pull up your sleeves.

THE GOOD MAN:
GEORGE WASHINGTON, FIRST PRESIDENT

The father of our country was not glamorous. Nor did he tear through the ladies of Paris the way his pal Ben Franklin did. But quietly, moderately, with great strength and honesty, he stayed the course during the war with England, displaying his doubts only to close friends. You could be GW. Maybe. It's hard to be a success on the battlefield and in the boardroom.

PRIMARY BENEFIT: You know what you do is good.

BIGGEST DOWNSIDE: You can't drool your deepest, darkest feelings all over others.

HOW TO KNOW IF YOU'RE THIS LEADER: While others worry about themselves, you inexplicably obsess about the organization and its people.

THE MONSTER:
JOSEPH STALIN, USSR DICTATOR

Stalin believed himself to be the inventor of every good idea. Those who did what he wanted had a better chance of staying vertical than those who didn't, but in the end just about everybody who came near him bought the gulag. You don't want to be like him. Of course, if you are, nothing I can say will dissuade you.

PRIMARY BENEFIT: It's fun playing with spleens.

BIGGEST DOWNSIDE: You must be very angry all the time, even while sleeping.

HOW TO KNOW IF YOU'RE THIS LEADER: When you see a puppy, you imagine it in a sandwich.

THE HUNGRY GUY:
BILL CLINTON, 42ND PRESIDENT

Bill Clinton is actually pretty simple.

He's a wonk and a grind and always studies every aspect of an issue, which is why he can talk for hours about anything. He has a big lust for the things a man should lust for: fame, power, ribs. And, of course, he's a numbnuts when it comes to women. Oh, and he has a tendency to say what's necessary to make problems go away, which makes him just like every business executive I've ever known, including myself. Personally, I think you could do worse than Bill Clinton. But if you're a Republican, fine, lead like Ronald Reagan. Charm and power make a great combination.

PRIMARY BENEFITS: There are new ideas, terrific foods, and women gathering round you.

BIGGEST DOWNSIDE: People hate men who can't control Mr. Johnson.

HOW TO KNOW IF YOU'RE THIS LEADER: You want what you want, and you just don't care.

THE BRILLIANT NUTCASE: HOWARD HUGHES, BUSINESSMAN

Hughes was never wrong, even when he was—a quality you must have to be a world-class boss. Hughes was also a bona fide nut. He was so afraid of germs he refused to shake hands (as does Donald Trump) and had special tactics for opening his dietary staple: canned peaches. You crazy enough to be him?

PRIMARY BENEFITS: Amazing wealth, unimaginable power, great hotel accommodations.

BIGGEST DOWNSIDE: Must deal with munching hedgehog floating in the air behind you.

HOW TO KNOW IF YOU'RE THIS LEADER: You see incredible strategies before anyone; little men in funny green suits dance for you at night.

YODA: STEVE JOBS, CEO, APPLE, INC.

Are you smart, cool, and in tune with the cosmos to a frightening degree? Then reach for this paradigm. Sure, it's like saying you'll work on being Buddha or Sir Isaac Newton or Thomas Edison, but why not? We need more guys like you.

PRIMARY BENEFIT: You see the world in a paper cup.

BIGGEST DOWNSIDE: You commute to work from Planet Mambo.

HOW TO KNOW IF YOU'RE THIS LEADER: You see people's lips moving, but what they say sounds like baboons grunting.

THE SCIENCE OF AMBITION

ONE LEVEL OF PERSONAL DRIVE IS MOST LIKELY
TO PRODUCE TRUE SUCCESS. AT THE OTHER EXTREME IS
THE LEVEL THAT WILL RUIN YOUR LIFE, OR KILL YOU.
WALK THE LINE BETWEEN THE TWO

BY LAURENCE GONZALES

I once traveled with the Penske Racing Team—the guys who won the Indianapolis 500 13 times. I wanted to find out how, and why.

Reason number one was fairly obvious: Roger Penske's testosterone overload. The higher your testosterone level, the less you use language, and the more you rely on action to speak for you. Penske, clearly the alpha male of his team, was practically mute. Al Unser Sr.'s wife, Karen, told me, "Roger talks in half sentences. He'll just be getting to the point, and he'll turn around and walk away."

The general manager of the team, an affable, intense Scotsman named Derrick Walker, told me, "When R.P. walks away, the ground is smoking." Walker's responsibility was to coordinate a team of cracker-jack mechanics to make sure the car was ready for the race. On R.P.'s team, "ready" meant ready to win. Or, as Walker put it, "Roger loves to go to the track and just blow their doors off." In contrast to Penske's testosterone levels, Walker's seemed manageable. He was fluid, helpful, cooperative, and diplomatic.

Of course, neither Penske nor Walker did the actual driving. They relied on a mild-mannered, soft-spoken, gently smiling guy named Rick Mears. He looked like a high-school English teacher who'd wandered onto the track. At about 150 pounds, he was slight and wore soft brown corduroy pants, a brushed-cotton shirt, and Top-Siders. In contrast to both Penske and Walker, Mears never seemed to hurry, never made abrupt movements. I watched him drinking one night after he'd been driving at well over 200 miles an hour all day, and even his drinking was like that: sip after sip, beer after beer, never off the pace.

These three men represented the height of ambition and success, yet they were very different from one another. Penske was clearly in charge, but he was contained within himself and his own obsessive thoughts of dominance. Walker was deferential to Penske, but he was just as clearly the boss of his team of mechanics. He was more open to the world, figuring out ways to enlist people to help him. Walker smiled a lot. Penske did not. Mears, on the other hand, was the one who stepped into the spotlight. Yet he deferred to both Walker and Penske.

In this way, they were very much like the hierarchies that other primates—chimpanzees, for example—set up in nature. This dynamic is afoot in many workplaces, where the boss might be the most dominant guy in the place, and also the most vulnerable. His lieutenants serve him, but they also benefit from the cover they get by being farther down the flowchart. So, just where is the sweet spot? Look to the Penske team for an indicator. Mears would have been miserable in Penske's shoes. And Walker, who built and prepared the car, didn't have the temperament to drive it. They were three natural prototypes for ambition, success, and dominance in the human world. And what they can teach us is that true success is possible on several levels of a hierarchy.

Being the alpha male—the one who feels the call to dominate and allows nothing to stand in his way—comes with tremendous costs. "We call them coronary-prone, type-A personalities," says Dean Simonton, PhD, a professor of psychology at the University of California at Davis. "They have extremely high stress, leading to nervous breakdowns or uncontrolled rages."

There are upsides, too, and not just in the paycheck. "The unambitious are the pawns of fate," says Dr. Simonton. "The ambitious make their own fate. And the triumph in accomplishment can be an awesome joy."

Sam Walton, founder of Wal-Mart, made that a lifelong pursuit. When he was in the hospital, dying of cancer, he had one last wish: to work some more. Only when store managers would stop by to visit him would he perk up, peppering them with questions about what they could do to improve the already astronomical bottom line. Like Penske, Walton was a deadly competitor. He opened his first Wal-Mart in 1962 and eventually grew to be the richest man in the world (a title he held until Bill Gates built Microsoft).

PERCENTAGE THE AVERAGE WORKING GUY RECEIVED FOR HIS LAST RAISE:

7.4

There have to be Penskes and Waltons in this world. But extremes don't necessarily lead to happiness or fulfillment. Neuroscientists, such as Gregory Berns, MD, PhD, of Emory University, in Atlanta, Georgia, have shown that fantastical sums of money won't make us happy, because the feeling we identify as satisfaction comes only when we anticipate a reward or triumph, not when we achieve it. The best way to keep this system working is to take up new challenges, especially ones in which you might fail.

But here's an interesting twist to the system: Philip Brickman, a former social psychologist at Northwestern University in Chicago, found that people who had been in an accident serious enough to cripple them enjoyed life no less than everyone else. In the same famous study, he determined that lottery winners were actually happier before their windfall.

In other words, the way our brains work makes it possible for us to get used to—and eventually even dismiss—anything. And if we're ambitious, then when something new and interesting happens, whether it's success or failure, our satisfaction meter is reset, and we start striving all over again.

The comedian George Carlin once said that the trouble with cocaine was that it made him feel like a new man. "And the new man wanted some." Ambition makes us that new man, because renewing our pursuit is the only way to experience the feeling of satisfaction—of success anticipated—again. Okay, we're junkies, but junkies for success.

By any measure, my friend Michael Mauboussin is both ambitious and successful. He played soccer, ice hockey, and lacrosse in school. He had no idea what he wanted to do for a living, though he was smart and did well in school. Just out of Georgetown University, he took a job at Drexel, Burnham, Lambert as a retail broker and began working his way up. He could have been an ordinary drudge, like most of his young peers, except for one thing: Michael wanted to do something big. Something difficult and different. He had his eyes open for an opportunity. He wanted something more and wanted it faster.

He started out as a junior analyst at Nomora Research Institute

America, gathering information about stocks for his boss to include in his reports. But he began spending evenings and weekends analyzing stocks that his boss wasn't covering, and writing the reports himself. They went out under somebody else's name, but Michael was doing the work of a senior analyst for no other reason than that he chose to. It was an intoxicating feeling. "That was an incredible learning phase," he says. He was in search of something he could not name. He was creating himself on the fly.

AMOUNT THE AVERAGE WORKING GUY THINKS HIS BOSS IS WORTH A YEAR:
$120,496

AMOUNT THE AVERAGE WORKING GUY THINKS HE SHOULD BE MAKING A YEAR:
$91,623

In his spare time, Michael read all the financial books he could get his hands on. That's how he stumbled onto Alfred Rappaport's groundbreaking book *Creating Shareholder Value*, which flew in the face of everything stock analysts—including Michael's boss—thought they knew at the time. For Michael, it was a new way of looking at stocks and how to set their value. Moreover, it was what he'd been looking for: a way to distinguish himself from everyone else. It was, he knew, a piece of the mysterious puzzle he was working out.

What he was doing at an almost instinctive level was making a series of decisions as he moved through life, like a basketball player moving the ball down the court. These decisions were carried out (for the most part unconsciously) through circuitry in his brain that had been honed to take in cues from the environment, interpret their meaning, and act on that meaning. In performing these maneuvers, Michael was manipulating the workings of an area in the brain called the striatum, which is the central gateway that combines thought, gut feelings, emotions, and hard information. When you're trying to drive through a busy intersection, your striatum is feathering the gas pedal, deciding when to punch it. With the added nitro fuel of testosterone, your instinct is turned into action. The higher your testosterone level, the more likely you are to hit

AMOUNT THE AVERAGE WORKING GUY MAKES A YEAR:

$57,816

the gas when there's barely enough time to get across ahead of that Lexus SUV. The reason we take such chances is not because getting hurt feels good. It's that the chance of getting hurt makes not getting hurt feel better. And that phenomenon lies at the core of our ambition.

For much of the 20th century, scientists thought that once the brain had developed in childhood, it contained a fixed number of neurons with immutable connections. The adult brain didn't change, they said. In recent decades, scientists have recognized that view as wrong: The brain—indeed, the entire organism—is remarkably plastic. Not only do we create our brains and selves through the experiences we have while growing up, but we continue to create ourselves throughout our lives. The psychologist Edward Taub showed how malleable the brain was when he taught stroke patients to use their paralyzed limbs, which was thought to be impossible at the time. But to remap the brain takes effort. You have to want it.

Where does drive like that come from? For that matter, why do we do anything at all? The answer is that a chemical in the brain called dopamine creates a will to act. Dr. Berns calls it "a chemical of anticipation" and points out that satisfaction is found not in achieving a particular goal but in working toward it.

To some extent, we're born with our own set level of ambition. Some of us come into the world grabbing for all we can get, active, competitive, aggressive, hungry for learning. Others are content to take table scraps. And in between are all shades of ambition and dominance. Those differences reflect the varying levels of dopamine and testosterone we produce.

Testosterone plays a crucial role in ambition. Those who have more of it have larger amygdalas, where aggression lurks, waiting to lash out. The high-T guys fight more and breed more. They have a more intense focus on work, are more persistent, and may be just plain stubborn. Men with high testosterone levels smile less and talk less. They also tend to go bald early, to maintain less body fat, to be self-confident, and to act up and act out more often. Football players, rattlesnakes, and stallions all have high testosterone. Everyone has a different level of the hormone, inherited from his parents. But the level rises and falls depending on all sorts of factors, from the season of the year to whether we win

AMOUNT OF MONEY THE AVERAGE WORKING GUY WOULD NEED PER YEAR TO LIVE WORRY-FREE:

$133,517

or lose at any activity. (Testosterone varies in women, too; female lawyers have more of it than female nurses do.)

The brain chemistry that goes into generating the drive to perform is extremely complex, and we're only beginning to understand it. But the importance of testosterone and dopamine is not in dispute. As important as ambition is, there are surprisingly few cells that produce dopamine, about 30,000 in all. The richest area for dopamine activity is the striatum, located in the brain stem, where notions are turned into action. Those of us who have a robust striatum, plentiful dopamine, and a reasonable level of testosterone learn early on what William Butler Yeats called "the fascination of what's difficult." The striatum is most active when, say, your boss stands in your door and offers you an opportunity that sounds vaguely like a threat.

"Cortisol [the stress hormone] is released when an individual's active pursuit of some reward is jeopardized by events," says Oliver Schultheiss, PhD, an associate professor of psychology at the University of Michigan. That triggers a hormonal cascade of adrenaline, with a testosterone and dopamine chaser. You cue up your brain and body to take on new skills, says Dr. Schultheiss, and do it quickly before something dire results: "The punishments include death, pain, loneliness, and low status."

The outcome is unclear, which is just the thing to send your hormones, and achievement, into overdrive.

Not surprisingly, financial managers have 24 percent higher testosterone than others in the business, according to James McBride Dabbs, PhD, a psychologist who has made a career studying the levels of this chemical in various professions. After reading *Creating Shareholder Value*, Michael Mauboussin immediately put theory into practice, writing up a report on Ralston Purina stock using the radical new technique. "I handed a draft of my report to my senior analyst, and he read it and sort of flicked it back at me and said, 'This will be of minor academic interest, but no one in the real world will ever care about it.'"

That was a crucial moment for the 26-year-old junior analyst in his first real job. It could have gone quite differently if he had taken his superior's advice and returned to analyzing stocks the conventional way. But instead, he felt his old athletic competitiveness kick in. The robust dopamine system told him, "This is hard. This is new. This is different." The possibility of failure meant that it might just be very rewarding. In addition, engaging in any sort of risky activity increases the transient level of testosterone in the bloodstream. (Firefighters on the way to a fire have high testosterone. On the way back, their levels fall considerably.) Michael's testosterone system was alerting him to the fact that this was a test of dominance, too. He sent the report out as it was and waited for the response.

"My thinking was, Maybe this won't work, but I'm going to go down trying like crazy." Without knowing why at the time, Michael was doing what people with well-functioning striatal and testosterone systems do: He was selecting the course of action that held the chance of the most satisfying experience, where novelty but not success was guaranteed.

Neuroimaging studies have shown that predictable rewards do not activate the striatum or produce dopamine and testosterone nearly as well as unpredictable rewards do. To succeed, you have to be willing to fail. As John F. Kennedy said when exhorting the nation to send men to the moon, "We choose to do things not because they are easy but because they are hard."

The report from Michael's big brokerage firm went to a select list of clients, and a few weeks later, the chairman of Ralston Purina, Bill Stiritz, one of the smartest guys in the industry, invited Michael out to St. Louis to share his views with the top executives. If Michael's life had been a movie, this is where he would leap up from his desk, fist in the air, and say, "Yesss!" He had just bodychecked his boss on the ice, and it was the beginning of an enormously successful career that today finds him at the top of his field. But, even more important than that,

Michael is doing what he loves and living a life he thoroughly enjoys, with a kind of freedom that most people only dream about. He had to work hard when he was starting out—but not gruesomely hard. He put in 10-hour days and perhaps half of Saturday at the office, then had time to play some pickup basketball. He worked out at the gym. He married his college sweetheart in 1990, and as they took on the responsibility of their first child in 1993, he gradually began to carve out more and more time for his home life.

"I don't know that you can be productive working 90 hours a week," he says. "I'm always working in the sense that I'm always thinking and reading. But there has to be some sort of balance." In other words, his drive did not turn him into a Roger Penske or a Sam Walton.

And this suggests that Michael has another key ingredient in what may be the most rewarding kind of ambition and success: serotonin. This chemical works in some of the same areas that testosterone does but tends to give people an agreeable deportment. Serotonin mellows out the effects of testosterone and may in fact reduce levels a bit. Guys with high serotonin are cool and confident, optimistic, and generally more pleasant to be around.

While it's true that alpha males like Walton and Penske succeed and enlist followers by brute force, they are anything but cool and comfortable. They're on the ragged edge of a never-ending emergency. Most people like to associate and work with those who make them feel good. That's one reason dominant, successful men don't necessarily have high testosterone. If they have enough testosterone and sufficient serotonin, though, they have a winning combination of aggressiveness, competence, calm, and a smile that enlists support from men and admiration from women.

According to the psychiatric researcher Jeffrey Schwartz, MD, of the UCLA school of medicine and author of *The Mind & the Brain*, when the striatum is working normally, it coordinates enormous amounts of information, much of which we're not even aware of, and translates that into complex, coordinated actions. The striatum receives information from the rational, thinking part of the brain (the cortex) as well as the emotional part of the brain (the limbic system) and includes what researchers refer to as "error-detection circuitry," or "the worry circuit."

Along with a man's personal drivetrain, involving the striatum, dopamine, serotonin, and testosterone, this provides a crucial modulating device for directing our actions in the world: You have to not only know and strive for what's going to benefit you, but know what's bad for you and avoid or correct it. In some people, this "worry circuit" malfunctions—or functions too actively—and in extreme cases, this can lead to obsessive-compulsive disorder. In those annoying office guys who read Sun Tzu and eat razor blades for breakfast, it leads to simply trying too hard.

Like the fluid and seemingly effortless way a great skier carves down the mountain—avoiding danger and gaining velocity on the fly—people with a good balance among these systems will move through life with grace and ease, dodging difficulties and embracing challenges. I think of Michael Mauboussin's success that way. *SmartMoney* magazine named him to its "Power 30" list as one of "the most influential people on Wall Street." The perfect mix of dopamine, testosterone, and serotonin put him there.

In trying to explain how he became as successful as he is, the only thing Michael can point to directly is his penchant, encouraged by a mentor he sought out, the legendary Bill Miller, for educating himself in diverse fields of knowledge. As a member of the board of trustees of the Santa Fe Institute, Michael reads everything from quantum mechanics to neuroscience and history. As Dr. Berns puts it in his book *Satisfaction*, "People who seek out information about the world get more goodies. . . . Far from curiosity killing the cat, the need for novelty has made us who we are—intelligent, curious, and constantly seeking the next new thing."

In many ways, then, it appears that we're handed our ambition when we receive our genetic package. Some of us will be driven, some not. But here's an interesting thing about the striatum and the dopamine system: It's activated by many changes in the environment. The expectation of something good will activate it, but so will an electric shock or a noxious smell. Pain activates it very effectively, perhaps to motivate you to find a way to make the pain stop. That's why running a marathon can be satisfying, even though it hurts, and why a miserable guy like

Johann Sebastian Bach could crank out tunes at such a prodigious rate. (His 20 children seem to suggest a high testosterone level, too.)

How we think about ambition and success has a lot to do with who we are and the natural gifts we're given when we come into the world. There are no born losers. But there are a lot of people who choose the wrong path or find themselves pushed there. You might, for example, become a doctor because that's what your father is, when in reality you hate practicing medicine and love fixing cars.

A variety of studies have shown that people who achieve extraordinary things need not be extremely intelligent. They're smart, with IQs of 120 or 130, but they're not too smart. As Nancy Andreasen, MD, PhD, a psychiatrist and clinical researcher at the University of Iowa, points out in her book *The Creating Brain*, what these extraordinary individuals do possess is a personality that is adventurous, rebellious, individualistic, playful, persistent, and curious. They tend not to be influenced by preconceptions and to go their own way with a sense of confidence, just as Michael did when people told him that his ideas about valuing stocks were wrong. High achievers' openness means that they try to see the world in fresh ways all the time. They're rarely looking at something and saying, "I can ignore that, because I already know what it's all about." They look again. And again. They always approach new situations with new curiosity.

In the early '90s, Penske noticed a loophole in the Indy 500 rules that allowed a push-rod engine to have more horsepower than a turbo engine. He developed a car based on this loophole and took everyone by surprise in the 1994 race, giving Mercedes its first win at Indianapolis since 1915. The rule was changed the next day, but the Penske team had bagged its 10th Indy 500.

People who achieve extraordinary things aren't put off by ambiguity. Michael went through a large part of his career not knowing where he was going. He says, "I never had a game plan whatsoever. I was just going to do what I thought was interesting and have fun doing what got me fired up." Such people also are natural explorers, compulsively curious; they push against rules and conventions. Michael deliberately

(continued on page 292)

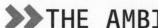

THE AMBITION PRESCRIPTION

8:00 a.m.: Beat Your Coworkers to the Punch

Start your workday bathed in the sickly glow of a gossip blog and you'll sabotage your productivity all day, says Julie Morgenstern, author of *Never Check Your E-mail in the Morning*. "When you accomplish a high-level task first thing in the morning, that sense of productivity feeds into the rest of your day," she says. These three quick fixes will optimize your first 60 minutes at your desk.

Lay the groundwork: Your workday really began in the last hour of the day before, when you contemplated the disaster zone known as your desk. "Never leave your office without knowing exactly what you're going to do with the first hour of the next day," says Morgenstern.

Hit a leadoff home run: "Use your brain's prime time for prime-time work," says Ronni Eisenberg, author of *The Overwhelmed Person's Guide to Time Management*. So, target one major project in your first hour on the job: Knocking it off early amplifies your efficiency once you start multitasking again. The brain is better at multitasking later in the day, anyway, after you've had a chance to wake up.

Tune out Outlook: "E-mail has created an instant-response culture," says Morgenstern. "It turns you into a reactive slave to Outlook." So turn off that "alert" noise, steal a "Do Not Disturb" hotel tag and post it prominently, and punch the "hold all calls" button on the phone. Now you're cooking.

9:00 a.m.: To Become Head Clown, Manage the Bozos

"Nowhere is it written that work is supposed to be fun. So you're going to have to deal with difficult people," says Alan Cavaiola, PhD, coauthor of *Toxic Coworkers*. Here's how to star among this very eccentric cast of characters.

The tattletale: Dwight Schrute (Rainn Wilson) on *The Office*: He's eager to make you a rung in his climb up the corporate ladder, so avoid a power struggle with him. "Focus your energy on improving relationships with high-level people," says Marie G. McIntyre, PhD, author of *Secrets to Winning at Office Politics*. If they respect you, then Dwight's sabotage attempts will expose him as the ass that he is.

The right-hand man: Smithers on *The Simpsons*: Use him as a conduit to the top. "The best interests of the organization matter most," says Rhona Graff, vice president and executive assistant to Donald Trump. "Let that person know what's being done—

and planned—in your department." Pitch projects and offer to head them up—then cc Smithers on all major developments. He'll keep the boss apprised of your progress.

The office psycho: Patrick Bateman (Christian Bale) in *American Psycho:* Don't try to defuse this time bomb. But don't ignore him, either. "Hear him out, but don't patronize him or try to fix his complaints," says Cavaiola. A bit of passive sympathy could save you from the shrapnel when the bomb finally blows.

The office gossip: Dennis Finch (David Spade) on *Just Shoot Me:* Avoid the chatty Finches; they're time wasters. Seek out the company's wise sages instead. "They know everything about the company," says McIntyre. "They can teach you the corporate culture and tell you how to make things happen."

The hottie: Veronica Corningstone (Christina Applegate) in *Anchorman:* Her assets will garner good assignments. So ask your boss for even better ones, says Dr. Cavaiola. Bosses will rarely turn down a request to do more. If Veronica still gets the plum projects, find an area of specialized knowledge and shape yourself into the company expert. Pecuniary interests usually trump prurient ones.

9:30 a.m.: Handle the Boss's Blast Like Jeter

What the boss says: "I need this ASAP."

What you should do: Drop everything. That said, most supervisors will have no idea of your workload, unless you keep them informed. So if his ASAP bomb hits your overloaded boat, give him your priority list and ask him where the latest salvo fits. He gets your timely execution and an education in your contributions at the same time.

9:45 a.m.: When You're Desperate for a Bright Idea, Genius Lurks Here

Don't be a cog. The way to move up is by generating creative solutions that exceed your employer's expectations. We assembled a panel of creative minds—from rappers to researchers—to help you hop any inspirational hurdle.

Hurdle: Your ideas are either too wild or too tame.

Solution: Use both sides of your brain. "The right hemisphere is more involved in the appreciation of novelty, but the left is needed for selection of utility," says Robert Bilder, MD, a professor at UCLA and a member of the Center for the Study of the Biological Basis for Creativity. The most innovative ideas involve both. Scribble all your creative ideas down on paper. Later, employ your utility detector to determine which ideas might earn you a promotion, and fill in the working details. Only then go to the boss.

(continued)

Hurdle: The pressure of generating impromptu ideas at the weekly brainstorming session leaves you overwhelmed and underrecognized.

Solution: Do your research. "I don't feel that I'm a natural at rapping, so I take the beat and study it," says Talib Kweli, a hip-hop artist and the former partner of Mos Def in Black Star. Kweli says he has to work to make his music happen. "I'm not good at writing hooks, so I have to work hard at that. I get into a song and go at it for weeks." Get your hands on the agenda the day before the meeting and develop your ideas. Claim a prominent seat at the meeting, so they know who the "new" guy is with all the brilliant ideas.

Hurdle: Your creative engine is running out of gas.

Solution: Refuel outside of the workplace. "Always be open to inspiration," says Al Jean, executive producer and head writer of *The Simpsons*, the longest-running sitcom in television history. "Great ideas come from everywhere, and it's important to follow up on them immediately, while they're fresh," he says. You'll know you're in the right profession, says Jean, when you become inspired by everyday situations. "When I look at people now, they have overbites and yellow skin."

10:30 a.m.: Cover Your Butt (with Glory)

What the boss says: "This thing could have legs. It'll be important for us to get buy-in from management."

What you should do: Stake your claim. Unlike 97 percent of what you do every day, this could actually go somewhere—provided the higher-ups agree with your boss. So shepherd all the niggling details your boss doesn't have time for. He'll need you in the presentation meeting—as a minutiae wrangler and ass coverer—so when the green light shines, it will bathe your face as well.

12:00 p.m.: Land a Much Better Job

Job interviews shouldn't feel like gladiatorial combat. The trick is to show that you already fit in while crisply handling awkward—but predictable—lines of questioning.

Q: Why should we hire you?

A: I produce results, and I have strong analytical skills and good initiative. Wouldn't you like to work with a manager with 3 years of experience in this position who's a breeze to get along with?

Why it works: The interviewer is looking for specific examples to help him or her evaluate how strong the candidate is, says Robin Kessler, author of *Competency-Based*

Interviews. Explain concretely how you fit that mold, and tell the tale of how an 11th-hour inspiration benefited a past employer. Managing deadline pressure is always a plus.

Q: What is one of your weaknesses?

A: I'd like to understand the nitty-gritty of technology better so I can use it to implement my best ideas.

Why it works: Forget the ploy of portraying a strength as a weakness (e.g., "I'm a workaholic"). Talk about a specific skill set you'd like to improve on. "Technology is ever-changing, and I'm looking for people who recognize the areas where they can seek more knowledge," says Laurie Minard, director of human resources at GPS manufacturer Garmin International.

Q: Why are you leaving your current job?

A: I feel like I've come a long way in the 3 years I've worked at Initech, but I think now is the right time for me to branch out into a new area.

Why it works: Trash-talking your old boss is a fool's game. "Every interviewer subconsciously sees himself as your potential ex-employer, whose faults will ultimately be broadcast to the world," says Paul Powers, PhD, author of *Winning Job Interviews*. Focus instead on how this new job will let you achieve successes you never would have reached in your old gig. You'll also show you're a motivated self-starter.

Q: What do you do in your off time?

A: I have a 3-year-old who keeps me on my toes. But I still shoot hoops on the weekends with friends, and I've been reading a lot about the Revolutionary War.

Why it works: "A new hire is someone you'll have to be around 40 hours a week for the next who-knows-how-many years, and it's almost like you get to hire a potential friend," says Mike Erwin, senior career advisor at www.careerbuilder.com.

4:15 p.m.: Manipulate Your Fate

What the bossman says: "Here's what I'm thinking, big picture—wise."

What you should do: Fill in the details. "This is your boss's way of making direct reports do all the actual work on a project," says Lois Beckwith, author of *The Dictionary of Corporate Bullshit*. So schedule a meeting with your boss, and force him to go over a specific plan of action with you. If he's invested in your work from the ground up, you'll have a better chance of succeeding and getting credit for it.

wanted to be different, what he calls a "tempered radical." He dressed in a suit and tie but was subversive in his ideas.

The adult brain, while slower to change than that of a child, is fully capable of changing in surprisingly dramatic ways, often in remarkably short periods of time. V. S. Ramachandran, MD, PhD, of the University of California at San Diego, was one of the first neuroscientists to demonstrate this conclusively in an adult. He obtained images of the brains of people who'd had an arm amputated and showed that the area that would normally receive sensation from the hand had been invaded by the nerves next to that area, which receive sensation from the face. As Dr. Ramachandran puts it in his book *Phantoms in the Brain*, "Brain maps can change, sometimes with astonishing rapidity."

So you can't exactly change who you are, but you can certainly change a great deal about yourself, including how smart, successful, and ambitious you are. For some of us, this will be like changing from being a smoker and 60 pounds overweight to running a marathon. For others, it will be more of what we're already doing.

History, if not science, shows that we don't do what we believe is impossible. It also shows that we can sometimes do what others consider impossible. In 1954, it was widely believed to be humanly impossible to run a mile in less than 4 minutes. Some people thought it would be fatal. Yet on May 6 of that year, Roger Bannister, then 25 years old, ran a mile in 3 minutes, 59.4 seconds. Within a couple of weeks, his record was broken, and it's been broken again and again ever since then, simply because people no longer believe it's impossible. In a variation on this theme, the famous supercomputer designer Seymour Cray said he hired kids right out of college, because they didn't know what the older engineers considered impossible, so they went ahead and did it.

What this means is that no one can give you a formula for success, for happiness and satisfaction in life. But knowing that it's possible to strive for that at any time—that the brain will go ahead and rewire itself if you insist that it do so—can be a powerful motivation to change. The dopamine, testosterone, and serotonin are locked and loaded, waiting for the call to fire. New challenges are the trigger.

WORDS OF THE UNWISE

NOTE THESE 11 THINGS YOU SHOULD NEVER TELL YOUR BOSS

BY GIL SCHWARTZ

I was sitting in a meeting the other day with quite a few guys whose ties probably cost more than your suit, and somebody said something that really frosted my oyster. A few years ago, I might have let it slide, but I'm relatively secure in my employment in this gulag, so out of my mouth flew "Jeez, Brad, that's total crap." Except I didn't use the words "jeez" and "crap," but I did employ two carefully selected four-letter words.

My point is, when it comes to what spews from your mouth at the office, you don't have to go tiptoeing around, worried about every word or phrase. That can actually be bad for your reputation as a smart shooter. The exception to this rule, however, is when you're talking to your boss. With him, there are certain statements that only a dunderhead would allow to pass his lips. And they are:

"YOU KNOW, ALAN, YOU NEVER TOLD ME TO DO THAT"

Employees who require specific orders to do valuable things are a total pain to the men who pay them. Okay, perhaps Alan didn't think of the precisely correct action and issue a formal request. So what? You want to remind him of that? Pointing out a boss's failure to think, act, or issue commands in any way is serious business. Besides, just because he didn't tell you to do it doesn't mean you shouldn't have known he wanted it done.

"NO CAN DO, RON. I'M JUST TOO BUSY"

Of course you're too busy. You're supposed to be too busy. Bosses hate when employees say they're too busy. We don't care. You don't want to

PERCENTAGE OF MEN WHO ADMIT TO THINKING ABOUT WORK DURING SEX:

14

be too busy? Get out of here. And don't you dare tell us that you can't start on project D until you've finished projects A, B, and C. If you can't multitask, we'll find somebody who can, or at least somebody who's willing to lie about it.

"BUT YOU GAVE ME THE EXACT OPPOSITE ORDERS YESTERDAY"

You fool! Of course he did. Bosses contradict themselves all the time, especially when they don't know what to do, and they really hate that feeling. They think one thing. They think another thing. They're not sure which is better, so they try both, or either, or neither, flailing around until they settle on the right course of action. What they want from their people is a free, nonjudgmental willingness to go with their flow without demanding that hobgoblin of little minds: consistency. This doesn't mean you should stop protecting your boss from his own confusion. Just be strategic: "You know, I'm working to find the interface between yesterday's approach and today's new angle. Help me with that for a minute."

"HEY! DON'T YELL AT ME"

He can yell at you if he wants. The silent Zen approach to being yelled at is better than the anguished outcry of a little baby. Staring is okay. Dignified moping, even. But hollering back? Highly inadvisable.

"YOU KNOW, BOB, I WAS AT A MEETING WITH CHUCK AND LENNY YESTERDAY . . ."

Don't even finish. What were you doing meeting with Chuck and Lenny? Conspiring against Bob? Well, that's what it sounds like, Judas. And who made them so smart all of a sudden? Bosses hate being talked about behind their backs, being shown up by colleagues who just might have better ideas than they do, or feeling that you're just as willing to work with others. If you've been having legitimate meetings with others on matters of importance, just let your boss know what the ideas were and ask for his thoughts on them.

"ACTUALLY, PAUL, I'M NOT MUCH OF A TENNIS PLAYER"

True story: A few years ago, I had this friend in the company, Joe. And Joe was a great sportsman. He golfed. He swam. He rode a big hog. Very cool dude. So one day the chairman of the corporation, about 16 grades above my pal in the hierarchy, gives him a call. The Big Dog is actually on the line! "Hey, Joe," says the chairman, very palsy-walsy. "I understand you're a runner. So am I. You want to run together some morning?" And Joe, for reasons I will never understand, says, "Actually, Paul, I like to run in the afternoons." "Oh," says the chairman, bruised and nonplussed. "Okay, then. See you sometime." And that is the last time Joe ever spoke with the chairman.

"THAT'S NOT MY JOB"

Oh, I see. You have a job description, do you? No, you don't! The only job description worth anything is the one that says, "Do whatever you need to do to make your boss think that without you, his life would suck." That's your job description. I can't tell you how many times I've made a mental note to torture some lazy, resentful turd who told me this or that essential thing wasn't his job. In fact, now that I think of it, nobody around here has said that for a really long time. Know why? All the people who have said it, or were perhaps likely to say it, are now at home in their pajamas.

"I GOTTA GO HOME. I'M TIRED"

Huh? You're tired? Men don't get tired. Men march and march and march the entire length of China for their leader! Okay, not every boss can inspire that kind of loyalty (and fear), but it is always and inevitably at the exact worst moment that people get to the end of their ropes and start collapsing. Be tired when there's nothing going on—when everybody is bored on a summer Wednesday, maybe, or on a snowy Friday right after New Year's. But when everyone around you is losing it, maintain. Your boss is the one, in the end, who will decide when you're tired enough to call it quits.

"IF YOU DON'T GIVE ME THAT RAISE, I'M QUITTING"

I personally know at least three men who issued this old tomato and were immediately told, "Fine. Get out of here." You might get the same response if you're thinking about conjuring up a mythical offer from a rival firm, one that must be matched or else. Bosses don't like the whole "or else" thing. They're likely to be irrational about it. You, my friend,

▶▶FIVE THINGS YOU SHOULD NEVER SAY AT THE OFFICE

No matter how great your rage, don't let these gems pass your lips.

"My boss is in over his head." The boss hears everything—good or bad. "Assume what you say about him will get back to him," says Marie McIntyre, PhD, author of *Secrets to Winning at Office Politics*. "So if you need to vent, gripe to someone outside of work."

"Giddings is an idiot." Office gossip can unite the gossipers and foster communication, up to a point. But taken too far, gossip can also breed paranoia and cut productivity, says Bob Burg, coauthor of *Gossip*. Burg suggests deploying only useful information. As in, "Giddings bungled the deal because he didn't know his audience."

"If I can just push out Fishman . . ." The golden rule of corporate politics: Never reveal your entire strategy to anyone. Your boss should know that you want his job, but not that you're scheming to start next month. If you tell a workmate, the plot is vulnerable.

"I studied barbiturates in college." That night you spent in the hoosegow for public urination is a great story, but keep it to yourself. "Whatever you tell people now will become more widely known the higher you go in the organization," says Leslie Gaines-Ross, author of *CEO Capital: A Guide to Building CEO Reputation and Company Success*.

"Callihan got canned because of his body odor." Unloading embarrassing details about another employee undermines your credibility. "Always bring it back to business, and don't ruminate on the person's faults," says Burg. So make it, "Callihan didn't present the right image to clients."

—SARAH BALDAUF

are fungible, no matter how much you may believe you are not. His self-respect (or, if you prefer, arrogance) as a boss is not. If you put him in a position in which he must either fold or kill you, he will kill you. Would you expect anything less from him?

PERCENTAGE OF MEN WHO ADMIT TO THINKING ABOUT SEX DURING WORK:
98

"I'M SURE YOUR CONCERNS ARE COMPLETELY OVERBLOWN"

Bosses are paranoid for good reason: People are out to get them. So don't pooh-pooh his obsessive fears and delusions. They won't stop bothering him simply because you say they will. A boss is defined, in large part, by the things that worry him. Keep him company with his demons or he'll find someone who will.

"I LOVE YOU, MAN"

There are things that, once said, cannot be unsaid. Do you really want that kind of glop hanging around in the air between you forever? Show him you care in other little ways. In fact, I bet you already do every day, you big softie, you.

THE FIRING-SQUAD SURVIVAL GUIDE

BULLETPROOF YOUR CAREER IN SEVEN EASY STEPS

BY GIL SCHWARTZ

Most careers have expiration dates stamped on them. Guys come into the place all fresh and crispy. They stay that way for a while. Then they begin to droop a bit, turn a little funky around the edges. Before long, they're totally wilted and ready for the Dumpster.

It happens to just about all of us, no matter how smart or fast we might be. A lot of the time, it's nobody's fault. Bosses change. Business shifts. Jerks and predators take their toll. Even the quickest antelope on the veld eventually loses a step and becomes prey to hyenas of one sort or another.

There are a few, though, who beat the odds. Guys who seem to go on forever, like Dave Matthews jams. What do they have that others don't? A mastery of the seven rules of fireproofing. Now you'll know them, too.

RULE 1: KNOW THY BOSS

The most critical part of self-preservation is, of course, to perform your duties with distinction. If you don't, you can brush off your résumé right now, because you're going to need it every couple of years. But if you're great at what you do, a successful campaign for longevity begins with your ability to know the boss, serve the boss, please the boss, and become absolutely necessary to the well-being of the boss.

When he wakes up in the morning with a throbbing head, your boss should be able to think, I'll give that to Webster, assuming you, of course, are Webster. When he feels sad, this thought should immediately occur to him: Perhaps I should have a drink after work with Ned, assuming, likewise, that you are Ned. When I was starting out in corporate America, I played a sort of demented, inebriated Santa Claus at the chairman's private Christmas party every year. I'm convinced that I survived at least one horrible downsizing because he needed me come yuletide.

RULE 2: KNOW THY NEXT BOSS

Bosses are disposable, too, as tragic as that seems to those of us who invest so much time and affection in them. That boss whom I served as Santa for nearly 10 years one day woke up to find that the company had sold our unit. There was a new job for him in a part of the operation in which none of us had any interest, and that was it for him and me. If I had positioned myself as solely his guy, I would have been as thoroughly toasted as he was, though slightly less lucratively.

But, during his tenure, I had done what I always like to do: dropped by offices with coffee cup in hand, hung with the homeboys up and down the hallways, and paid respect to an entire cadre of senior officers who might one day rise to greatness and be of use to me.

Among that group was a fellow I'll call Bud. Bud was a bit of a loner, slightly off center, not very popular with the rest of the squad.

I liked him. He had a tendency to go off on huge flights of fancy, to imagine what would happen if we merged with Microsoft or the government of Tasmania. And when the Boss was sucked up and out of the enterprise, it was Bud whom the organization tapped to take the top job, simply because he was the craziest visionary in the building. And the first person he called to ask what to do? Me, of course. A year later, I was one of only four people who survived the change of power.

RULE 3: KNOW THYSELF

It's all very well to play with the big dudes in the flowing white robes who work in the ethersphere. Behind that, you have to have a working knowledge of you—who you are, what you can do, where you want to go, who you love, who you hate. In a business life, the one true tool of importance is you.

If you're reading this, you probably have a certain amount of ambition. Nobody without drive bothers to think about the strategies behind what we do; they just go through the motions, collect their paychecks,

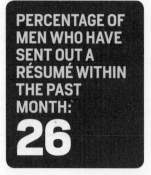

PERCENTAGE OF MEN WHO HAVE SENT OUT A RÉSUMÉ WITHIN THE PAST MONTH:

26

and hammer back brewskies at quitting time. The study of oneself may be the most important single effort you can undertake in your career. It never stops. It never grows old. You never stop benefiting from it—or hurting from the time you spend not doing it.

There's a classic line in the Clint Eastwood movie *Magnum Force*. Right after he blows somebody away, Clint mutters, "A man's gotta know his limitations." Engrave it on your desk.

There was this midlevel guy I know. Call him Wager. He was pretty good at whatever it was he was supposed to be doing. Everybody kind of liked him, but he didn't know his limitations. Whenever there was a job to do, he sucked it up. Whenever there was a meeting, he insisted on being there.

One day, the chairman wanted to meet to discuss something of interest to him—which meant something of very little interest to anybody else at that moment. Naturally, Wager had assumed responsibility for it. We all went to the meeting, which had international banking implications. Wager knew nothing about international banking. Afterward, the chairman pulled my boss aside.

"I never want to see that bonehead again," he said. And he didn't.

RULE 4: KNOW THY WORLD

Look around. If all you see is the tunnel to your office, the place you order your cheeseburger at noon, and the pipeline back home—with a possible bar or two in between—you're not taking in all the information you need to make yourself fireproof.

I don't know what business you work in, but unless you're an Amish laborer, my guess is that things are changing. Technology is exploding. All of a sudden, Google wants a piece of your lunch. Gigantic barns in India now perform the function formerly accomplished by two floors of people who used to be your neighbors before they lost their jobs and moved to India. All around you, guys are using buzzwords that were invented 5 minutes ago. What the hell is going on?

If you don't know, get smarter. It's the guys who can explain the brave new world to senior management whose potential departure turns the big boys' guts to cream cheese.

PERCENTAGE OF MEN WHO HAVE CHECKED JOB LISTINGS IN THE PAST 30 DAYS: 60

RULE 5: LOVE THY NEIGHBOR

You have to have friends. Players who spend all their time managing up will eventually be hung from their ankles by their peers.

Yes, bosses are important. Industry savvy is, too. But if you ignore the people who should be by your side, you'll be running down the halls with your hair on fire in no time. Why? Because nobody doesn't mess up. Nobody doesn't need help when he does mess up or when he needs to be prevented from doing so. The man who tries to be an island—to work only by sucking upward and hammering downward—will eventually be cast adrift when times grow funky. And they will, man. You can take that to the bank.

You make business friends by caring about the fates of other people. This may seem simple to you, but it's amazing how hard a job that is for a lot of successful men. Even if you don't feel all warm and fuzzy or have the slightest interest in anybody but yourself, make believe, dude. When the fat is exploding in your face and you need Larry and Barry and Chet to bail you out, you'll be very glad you did.

RULE 6: KILL THINE ENEMY

This shouldn't be too hard for you, once you get my permission. You have my permission. There. Isn't that a relief?

The great philosopher of power, Niccolò Machiavelli, prescribed death for assholes more than 500 years ago. He gave this advice to a prince who wished to remain in power. That's you. Machiavelli recognized that successful rulers eliminate their enemies by killing them dead. Not by exiling them. Not by negotiating with them or throwing them in prison or yelling at them in a very mean way. They take them out back and chop off their heads. Bam. Any reading of history reveals dozens of stories of supposed enemies who, allowed to live, came back and caused

trouble. It's not a nice part of ongoing success. But if you want to survive longer than the average operator, you'd best keep a couple of sharp
knives about your person.

That said, there are lots of ways you can kill somebody within a corporate framework. You can undermine him over a long period of time
with the key senior officers who care what you think. (You can bet he's
doing the same.) You can make sure he's not invited to key meetings in
your control. (You can bet he's doing the same.) And you can wait for the
proper moment to strike, and then do so, without guilt, hesitation, or
fear. (You can bet . . . well, you know.)

A world without jerks! That's what you're fighting for. Hang in there.
It's a marathon, not a sprint.

RULE 7: KEEP THINE EYES OPEN

Andy Grove, the former head of Intel and one of the great survivors,
pinpointed perhaps the key ingredient of a long career. "I believe in the
value of paranoia," he said. "Business success contains the seeds of its
own destruction. I believe that the prime responsibility of a manager is
to guard constantly against other people's attacks and to inculcate this
guardian attitude in the people under his or her management."

Does this sound like a happy way to live? Wouldn't it be better if we
could all just get along? Why can't long-term survival be based simply
on the jobs we do, instead of on all this political and military nonsense?

Good questions, all. Best of luck finding the answers. Until then, I'll
be around back, putting on my armor. See you there.

BE A BETTER DAD

The more time you spend with your kids, the better you'll be at your job. In a national survey of executives by www.theladders.com, an online recruitment service, 79 percent of respondents reported that being a father made them better professionals. "It's a career asset," says Stew Friedman, PhD, director of the Work/Life Integration Program at the University of Pennsylvania. "The skills men use to parent also help them manage their teams."

HAVE A COKE AND A NAP

If you're feeling drowsy at work, don't reach for a soda. British researchers discovered that people who downed a sugary drink containing 42 milligrams of sugar and 30 milligrams caffeine—the amount in a 12-ounce cola—exhibited slower reaction times and a greater number of lapses in attention for the next 70 minutes compared with those who sipped a sugar-free beverage. Although a sugar rush has been shown to boost cognitive performance, the effect is short-lived, lasting just 10 to 15 minutes. Your best option for a brain boost: a sugar-free drink that delivers at least 80 milligrams caffeine, says lead investigator Clare Anderson, PhD. A classic example: 8 ounces of black, unsweetened coffee.

Coffee does more than wake you up: Consumption of 6 to 7 cups a day is associated with a reduced risk of diabetes.

NUMBER OF MILES THE
AVERAGE WORKING
GUY IS WILLING TO
COMMUTE FOR A JOB:
34.6

GET ALL-DAY ENERGY

Sentenced to a day of hard labor? Bag the big lunch break. University of Montana researchers found that men work harder and longer when they eat small snacks all day long instead. In the study, wildland firefighters who grazed on small portions of easy-to-eat foods rested less and worked more during a 12-hour shift than when they ate the same number of calories in a large midday meal. Even if you're just cleaning the gutters, well-timed carbohydrate intake is key.

"Between 25 and 40 grams an hour provides your muscles with a constant fuel supply," notes study author Brent Ruby, PhD.

Here's some fast fuel: 2 ounces Planters Nut & Chocolate Trail Mix (27 grams carbohydrates), six peanut-butter-cracker sandwiches (25 grams carbohydrates), 16 ounces Gatorade (28 grams carbohydrates), Clif Builder's Bar (30 grams carbohydrates), large apple (29 grams carbohydrates).

POUR ON THE PERSUASION

Talk business at Starbucks and you might boost your sales. Australian researchers recently determined that a person is more likely to be persuaded if he's had a strong dose of caffeine. In the study, participants drank either the caffeine equivalent of two cups of coffee or a noncaffeinated placebo. Then they read a persuasive message on which they'd originally had an opposing opinion. The outcome: Caffeine drinkers were more easily swayed than those who downed none.

"Caffeine enhances alertness and concentration, enabling people to better evaluate the content of a message," says lead investigator Pearl Y. Martin, PhD. So pair a sound argument with a grande latte and you could have the formula to change a stubborn client's mind. If you use it to enhance your own powers of reason, choose a Starbucks Caffe Americano; it's loaded with caffeine, yet contains only 25 calories.

SCHEDULE RIGHT

Watch the clock to boost your brainpower. At certain times of the day, your brain is optimally prepared to do the most complex tasks, say doctors at the Sleep-Wake Disorders Center at Montefiore Medical Center, in the Bronx. To tap your brain's full potential, schedule your most challenging work for between 9 and 11 a.m. or 7 and 9 p.m. "That's when we're maximally alert," says sleep expert Michael Thorpy, MD.

TALK TO YOURSELF

It could keep you sane. A recent study by University of California researchers reveals that repeating a key word or two can slash your stress levels. When 66 people silently said a mantra—a meaningful word or phrase—during tense times, 83 percent felt less stressed. One critical point: People practiced their mantra first during calm moments, training their minds to associate it with relaxation. "A mantra can be used in brief snippets or for longer periods," says lead author Jill Bormann, PhD, RN. "It can be anything from 'shalom' to 'Take it easy.'"

BE ALERT TO THE LAST DROP

Perhaps on-the-job java should be a company mandate. Austrian researchers discovered that drinking a cup of coffee truly does make you mentally sharper. The scientists measured brain activity in 15 men

PERCENTAGE OF MEN WHO HAVE BEEN ASKED BY THEIR COMPANIES TO DO SOMETHING IMMORAL OR ILLEGAL:

11

after they consumed either 100 milligrams of caffeine—about the same amount as in a cup of joe—or a placebo. Test results showed that the caffeine group registered greater activity in the regions of the brain responsible for short-term memory, attention, and concentration. There's a time limit, though: The benefits diminish after 45 minutes.

CUT BACK

A University of North Carolina study links economic highs and low unemployment to higher fatal-heart-attack rates. Why? Long office hours lead to less exercise and more fast food.

MAKE A CRICK RECOVERY

If it feels like you're chained to your desk—by your neck—blame bad biomechanics. Typing without proper forearm support can cause chronic neck pain, reports a new University of California study. When researchers monitored 182 working stiffs for a year, they found that the people with forearm support were 50 percent less likely to have neck or shoulder pain than those left hanging. It's a domino effect: The weight of your arms pulls on your shoulder muscles, which drag on your neck.

Unfortunately, previous research shows that sitting in a chair with armrests won't help that much. "It might be because the armrests aren't the right height or are too far apart," says David Rempel, MD, the study's lead author. Instead, outfit your desk with a fixed forearm support, like the Morency rest (www.morencyrest.com). It was the device used in the study.

SIT, PRETTY

Is your job sabotaging your workout? Iowa researchers reviewed 15 studies that looked at the correlation between typing and disorders of the bones, joints, ligaments, tendons, and muscles. The study found that just 20 hours of keyboard use doubles your risk of hand and arm problems—and the chance of neck and shoulder disorders is even higher. The prescription: Keep your keyboard below elbow height, and type with your arms on armrests. This can improve posture and alleviate pain, the researchers report.

NUMBER OF MILES THE AVERAGE WORKING GUY IS WILLING TO COMMUTE FOR A JOB IF HE'S DRIVING A FERRARI:

50.2

APPLE MACBOOK PRO

Laptops are boring, so we'll keep this short. This is the fastest Mac ever (by far). It has a ton of smart features (like a magnetic power cord that snaps free when accidentally yanked). And because it's an Apple, you'll never have to understand how it works. (Brilliant.) ($2,000 and up. www.apple.com)

SONY READER

Most monitors and PDAs use flickering LCDs that tire your eyes. This e-reader shows flicker-free electronic versions of thousands of first-run books and graphic novels. The battery lasts through 7,500 page "turns," the 64 megabytes of expandable memory store up to 80 books, and the svelte ½-inch-thick package weighs less than four AAA batteries—even with the built-in rechargeable battery. Downside: It costs about 30 times the price of an actual paperback book. ($350. www.sonystyle.com)

SAMSUNG Q1 ULTRA-MOBILE PC

The first of the much-hyped ultra-mobile PCs, the Q1 can do anything your Windows laptop can—and it fits in your pocket. Its coolest feature:

a virtual thumb-driven keyboard that pops up on the 7-inch touch-screen. Built-in Wi-Fi lets you surf the Web and synchronize with your antiquated PC. (Price not set. www.samsung.com)

SLEEP PODS

In response to the millions of overworked, underrested employees of the world, MetroNaps has come up with a 20-minute solution—the $14 power nap. You repose in a state-of-the-art sleeping pod, which is a horizontal body-contoured chair fitted with a vibration device and Bose noise-cancelling headphones to help you nod off and sunrise-mimicking lights to help you wake up. Corporate zombies walk out feeling refreshed and even smarter. (Harvard researchers have proved that a 20-minute midday nap can enhance memory and boost productivity by up to 30 percent.) The company has locations in New York City and Vancouver, British Columbia. (www.metronaps.com)

MOTOROLA H5
MINIBLUE HEADSET

Bluetooth headsets make us feel like we're commanding the starship *Enterprise*. This one dials down the dork factor. Shove the pinkie-size stub in your ear and it automatically picks up your voice using the vibrations that run through your ear canal. That means no protruding microphones—and crisp, clear conversations even in the noisiest Klingon mess halls. (Price not set. www.motorola.com)

BEEF UP YOUR RAISE

FIVE WAYS TO GET WHAT YOU DESERVE

1. REMAIN CALM. It's okay to go Benicio Del Toro on the inside, but your face should remain Samuel Alito. "Unless the money is really good," says Dawson, "be grateful but not too eager." Tell your boss you need 24 hours to think about it.

2. TWELVE PERCENT IS THE MINIMUM. "It depends on the industry, but that's the average increase with a promotion," says Grazell R. Howard, president of the Libra Group, a consulting firm.

3. YES, THEY HAVE WRIGGLE ROOM. As a newbie to the position, you'll be offered a salary that's less than what your new peers are making. Savvy negotiators can use this knowledge to score a few thousand more. After you've thought about it for 24 hours, make your counteroffer. "If they've offered you 12 percent, ask for 18," suggests Dawson. "You'll most likely end up with 15."

4. ALWAYS ATTACK AGAIN WHEN THEIR GUARD DROPS. The point in the negotiation when your boss is most vulnerable, says Dawson, is when he thinks the negotiation is all over. "That's the best time to ask for perks like more vacation, an office, or a car service," he says.

5. NEVER LEAVE WITH NOTHING. A raise isn't in this year's budget? It happens. "Just make sure you have a clear agreement on when it'll go into effect," says Howard. When the time comes, hold your boss to it. And, as a reward for your patience and understanding, ask him to make it retroactive.

BURNING QUESTIONS

I love my family. I love my job. But sometimes my family and my boss both want more. How can I get a better handle on the two?

Start by creating some boundaries. The problem is that boundaries between work and family are so fluid that neither your boss nor your family knows what to expect, says Ellen Galinsky, president of Families and Work Institute, a nonprofit that conducts research on work-life balance. Sure, your boss sees the pictures of your kids and your wife on your desk, but you having a family is an abstract concept to a man who only sees you in a suit and tie. Your wife, for her part, probably thinks it's crazy that you can't ever get home by 6:00 to pick up your kids from soccer practice and have dinner as a family.

So establish some rules. Maybe it's that nothing will interfere with watching your daughter's Saturday soccer game, or that you'll come home each night to spend time with your family and then return to work once the kids are asleep. "Once your boss and your family know what to expect, no one will be surprised or upset," says Galinsky. "Just as important, you'll have worked out a compromise that you're happy with."

Of course, there will be times when you're faced with competing— and seemingly equally important—demands. Your boss might ask you to meet with clients the night of your wife's charity event, or your daughter's soccer final might conflict with a board meeting. In those cases, "Ask yourself this: A year from now, what will I wish I had decided?" says Galinsky. The average guy usually sides with work, spending only about a half hour a day taking care of his kids, according to the U.S. Bureau of Labor Statistics. Don't be average.

"Explain to your boss that you care very much about your company, but you have a prior engagement that you simply can't miss," says

PERCENTAGE OF MEN WHO SAY THEIR BIGGEST SOURCE OF STRESS IS WORK:

52

Galinksy. If he doesn't recognize the importance of family, then he's probably not a leader you want to commit yourself to long-term. But if there is a crisis at work and you simply can't attend a family event, do your job. You're a provider, after all, and to keep providing, sometimes you have to make compromises.

How can I get more done at work?

Forget the motivational books and try some scientifically tested tricks.

Remember the paperless office? Forget it. Print important e-mails and reports. Research shows that people are less likely to understand material or find it interesting if they read it onscreen, compared with on paper. And a stack of paper serves as a reminder.

Hang a picture of your mother-in-law—or any authority figure—on the wall. Researchers found that when a picture of human eyes hung over an honor box in a coffee room, people were more likely to pay in full than when a picture of flowers hung on the wall. "You behave more cooperatively when you think you're being watched," says Melissa Bateson, lead study author. "A picture of a face in your office will absolutely have a positive effect on your work behavior."

Get a second computer monitor. Researchers at the University of Utah found that adding a second screen helps you complete tasks 7 percent faster, makes you 10 percent more productive, and leaves you with 33 percent fewer errors. And 80 percent more likely to be beamed up to a corner office.

My e-mail gets crushed daily with spam. What's the best blocker?

Well, you're pretty much screwed, because we haven't found a spam filter that actually works. Short of purchasing anti-spam software, your best hope is to create a new primary e-mail address and give it out only to friends and family. Then use your old one for everything else, including online shopping. And remember, when it comes to spammers, never hit "unsubscribe." "That's the fastest way to let them know you exist," says Robert Vamosi, senior editor of software and services for CNET.

My boss seems to love useless meetings. Anything I can do at these gatherings besides daydream?

Absolutely. A productive meeting establishes what needs to be done, who will do it, and when. With that in mind, informally help your boss. You can also model productive behavior by asking good questions, being accountable and dependable, and respecting others' input. This should raise the energy in the room and gradually inspire others. Now, if the purpose of the meeting is to brainstorm ideas, then the what, who, and when aren't required. In those meetings, it's important to create an atmosphere where everyone's ideas are welcomed and seriously considered. Here, creative daydreaming is definitely okay.

My boss comes down on me any time I don't have a spreadsheet on my desk. How can I explain that I need breaks for my sanity and productivity?

Yeah, that's good—explain how stealing from the company helps the bottom line. Look, if you need to recharge, find a way other than going to YouTube for a chuckle. Walk to the john, go down the hall for an impromptu brainstorm in someone else's office, hell, take a walk around the building. Sitting at your desk doing nothing, no matter why you're doing it, only looks like one thing: like you're sitting at your desk doing nothing.

There's this jealous guy at the office who's chipping away at my reputation. I can't let him get away with it. How can I fight back?

There was this dude who used to play minor-league hockey—big beard, total goon. He was always ramming his glove under guys' chins, riding his stick in between their legs. Sometimes he got away with it, and sometimes he got clobbered. It may seem like you have only two choices—skate away or drop the gloves. But either of those extremes presents its own set of problems. Our thoughts: Careers are a contact sport, and if you feel like you're getting face rubs and nobody's calling a penalty, well, there's nothing wrong with returning the favor.

My boss is shady. I don't want to lose my job, but I don't want to go to jail, either. When do I have to squeal?

You aren't legally responsible for his shenanigans unless you knowingly help carry out a crime. But if he is committing crimes, continuing to work directly for him may put you in murky legal waters. There are laws that protect whistleblowers, so maybe it's time to speak up. Why stay as a deckhand on a sinking ship?

My boss often contradicts himself, which inevitably creates more work for me. How can I make sure that I understand him the first time?

If he's brilliant, suck it up, show an interest in how he arrives at the final decision, and learn from it. If he's reasonably intelligent but wishy-washy, ask him questions about possible alternatives from the get-go; that should help him clarify the reasoning behind each option and stick to one path. Then meet with him or request feedback at crucial junctures during the project. If he's just plain sadistic and derives joy from your suffering, find a new job.

An intern at the office is flirting with me like crazy. She'll be gone in a couple of months. Should I go for it?

You don't want to be the guy who hooked up with the intern. If the higher-ups catch wind of it—and trust me, they will—it'll put a dent in your professional reputation that could take years to hammer out. Besides, this girl is probably just using the same attention getting tactics in the office as she does at fraternity parties, because she doesn't know any better. Wait 2 months and hit on her as she's walking out the door.

PERCENTAGE OF MEN WHO SAY THEIR MOST EFFECTIVE STRESS RELIEVER IS SEX:
17

One of the higher-ups in the company talks trash about my boss when we're drinking. He also says great things about my future. Is there any way to play both sides?

Ever watch a baseball brawl? There are the guys who run out and jump on top of the pile, and there are the guys who stay on the fringes and bear-hug each other. Just because others are office-brawling doesn't mean you need to jump in. This higher-up may be baiting you, but nothing is more reassuring to a boss than a guy who's able to stay cool, respectful, and loyal, even when it's tempting not to. Keep yourself in good standing by accepting the compliments without throwing any punches.

I slept with my boss, but now I don't want to date her. What's my escape plan?

This is tricky. Say the wrong thing and the person in power may decide it's too embarrassing to have you around. You have to stroke this woman's ego as you extricate yourself. Tell her she's the ideal woman—beautiful, smart, sexy—then humbly insist that you couldn't possibly handle a relationship with someone you work with. Make it principle, not personal. As long as you don't fish off the company pier again next month, you should be in the clear.

Business stinks. How can I avoid getting canned?

Commence your defense. "Be sure to keep a current and very detailed list of all your achievements and contributions to the company so you can defend your position if need be," says Wendy

PERCENTAGE OF MEN WHO SAY THEIR BIGGEST SOURCE OF STRESS IS MONEY: 24

Enelow, a career coach and the author of *The Insider's Guide to Finding a Job*. "And always have an updated résumé ready to go, just in case." Book a meeting with your boss to learn about any new expectations he has, and to lay the groundwork for your future relationship. And stay in touch with old colleagues. You never know what opportunities they may have for you.

When I hit crunch time at work, my wife and I are at each other's throats. How do I get her to dial it back when work stress is at its peak?

Our guess is you're being shaken and shaken and shaken at work, and you're not telling your wife about any of it. Then, when the slightest bump hits at home, your emotional cork goes ricocheting off the walls. I don't think your problem is getting your wife to dial back. It's about letting off pressure so you don't pop.

I'm being promoted in a few months but have no information about my raise. How can I ask without sounding greedy or unappreciative?

C'mon, we know you want to look like you're more concerned with the company than the cash. But you're well within your rights to thank them for the promotion, tell them you're excited, then ask what kind of financial bump you can expect. In fact, if you don't, they might take you for a chump.

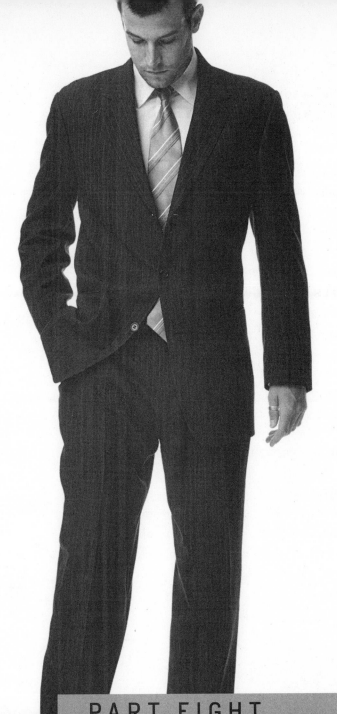

YOUR CLASSIC SUIT

CHOOSE THE BEST SUIT, COLLAR, AND CUFFS FOR YOUR MOST IMPORTANT MOMENTS

BY DAVID BEZMOGIS

Last year, a few months before my wedding, I planned to buy a suit. My intention was to go to Tom's Place, a men's store where I had, a year or two earlier, purchased a perfectly serviceable, single-breasted, navy blue Strellson suit. Tom's, true to its name, is owned by a man called Tom, who presides over a brigade of some 20-odd suit salesman. The store is located in Kensington Market, former hub of Toronto's immigrant Jewish vendors, and, though it stocks the likes of Boss, Cavalli, and Armani, it remains the kind of place where haggling is effectively encouraged. And whereas my wife-to-be had devoted months to the pursuit of a wedding dress, I planned to settle my business in a single leisurely trip to the market, ultimately walking away with a tuxedo or a sober black ensemble. The shopping experience would be, like most shopping experiences, a vaguely unpleasant imposition, essentially unremarkable but mercifully brief.

This was my plan, at least, until I spoke to my friend John, a television executive who spends more time in suits than I do. A suit or tux from Tom's was fine and adequate, he said, but was adequacy enough

**PERCENTAGE OF
MEN WHO DON'T
OWN A SUIT:
17**

for a monumental event like my wedding? John had had his wedding clothes custom made. Not only did the suit look and fit better, it, like the beginning of a new connubial life, was singular and pristine. If the idea appealed to me, he'd gladly take me to the shop where he'd just had a second suit made. The idea appealed to me, but I assumed that its appeal would be grossly mitigated by its expense. My frame of reference for such things was limited to a stroll past the exclusive shops of London's Jermyn Street and Savile Row. But John assured me that the price would be comparable to Tom's.

Now, when I say that John's idea appealed to me, I should clarify that it appealed to me only partly for the reasons he cited. Naturally I wanted a suit that looked good, and I could appreciate John's suit/connubial metaphor, but what attracted me was something altogether different and, I suppose, more esoteric: the desire to participate in a fading masculine tradition.

Literature and history attest to the fact that rich men, poor men, and military men all had their clothes custom made. Caravaggio, who was not renowned for his grooming or hygiene, liked to wear only the best materials and "princely velvets." Ulysses S. Grant, in his memoirs, recalled the eagerness with which he awaited his first uniform, ordered from a tailor immediately after Grant graduated from West Point. Even Mahatma Gandhi, famous for his white dhoti and shawl, once paid 10 pounds to have an evening suit made on London's fashionable Bond Street.

Until fairly recently, having a suit made was the rule rather than the exception. The experience was not always lavish, but even at its most humble, it reflected something ceremonial and dignified. In choosing to have a suit made, it was precisely this vestige of tradition and ceremony that I wanted to reclaim for myself—at least insofar as this was possible in Toronto, at the beginning of the 21st century, for under a thousand dollars.

John's suit came from a place called Acappella, a tidy, modern storefront run by a personable, somewhat boyish, well-dressed 34-year-old named Victor—a man who, for reasons having far more to do with pragmatism than nostalgia, had decided to offer his clients "made to measure" (MTM, in industry-speak). Victor, who ran the place with his father and brother, advised his clients on fabrics and styles and did the measuring. His technique wasn't strictly authentic, but for my purposes it sufficed. I wanted to avoid

NUMBER OF SUITS THE AVERAGE GUY OWNS: 1 or 2

another impersonal transaction as much as I wanted to be initiated into an old rite. This much, I believed, Victor could provide.

My initiation came in two stages: first, the selection of the fabric; second, the measuring. "Measuring," Victor told me, "is half the battle." Under his gaze, I sorted through fabric samples and isolated likely candidates. Along the way, Victor deciphered terminology. "One hundred percent wool." Now as ever, most suits begin as sheep. "Super 120." When a sheep is sheared, it yields longer filaments and shorter filaments. Longer filaments are woven into finer fabrics with more threads per cubic inch—hence, 120 threads per cubic inch. "Gabardine." Refers to the pattern of the weave. (A gabardine weave is diagonal. A grain weave is composed of tiny squares.) The fabric, like all the fabrics Acappella offers, originated in an Italian town called Biella, famous for its textiles. Thus, in a relatively short time, I was introduced to the history, origin, production, and classification of the material that would become my suit.

Having selected a fabric—100 percent wool, Super 120, black tone-on-tone striped gabardine—we proceeded to stage two. Victor placed me before a mirror, departed, and returned with the implements of the trade: a tape measure and two devices that were variations on the carpenter's level. These were prosaically called the "posture device" and the "shoulder device." Victor set the posture device against the back of my neck. Though I couldn't see it, I knew that a tiny bubble was traveling the length of a glass tube, coming to rest, and issuing a verdict on my posture: erect, regular, head forward, stooping, very stooping. Next came the shoulder device. A shoulder can vary anywhere from high to half high, regular, sloping, very sloping, and finally extreme sloping.

Some people, he explained, suffer from asymmetrical shoulders. No off-the-rack suits would ever properly fit such unfortunates; their only salvation lay in made to measure. My shoulders, Victor assured me, were symmetrical and regular.

As was my posture. Regular and regular. There was nothing wrong with me. Ludicrously, I felt relieved, happy, and proud, as if the label applied to more than just my posture.

The fitting concluded with the standard sequence of measurements: jacket length, sleeve, chest, half-back, outseam, inseam, waist, seat, knee, bottom. This was the part of the trade that had remained unchanged by time and technology. But Victor confirmed that this rit-

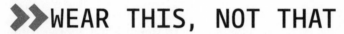

WEAR THIS, NOT THAT

The Collar

Choosing the right home for your knot no longer has to be a pain in the neck. The modern shirt collar hails from the tight-fitting frocks of the Elizabethan era, which is probably why most men think of them as male corsets. Here, *Men's Health* fashion director Brian Boyé offers some sartorial breathing room. "Not only should a collar never put you in a choke hold," he says, "but it should also harmonize the cut of your suit with the geometry of your face." There are dozens of collar styles to choose from, but we've narrowed it down to three basic choices. Follow the corresponding tips, and prepare to wipe off the lipstick.

OPTION 1: THE POINT

Recommended suit: Italian two-button peak lapel with side vents

Recommended knot: Four-in-hand or half Windsor

Who should wear it: A point collar is the go-to look for guys with round or square faces. Here's the rule: If your mug is massive, a narrow opening between the points of your collar balances the equation and makes for a more proportioned head shot. Once you have the right collar, it's critical to sport the correct tie knot. In this case, downsize. "Given the narrow opening," says Boyé, "you're defeating the effect with a thick knot."

You'll resemble: Robert De Niro in *The Untouchables*, Michael Douglas in *Wall Street*, and Cary Grant in nearly anything

ual's days were numbered. The old craftsmen, the last of their kind, were retiring, and replacing them—for all practical purposes—would be robots. Someone had already invented a machine called "the Fitter." Victor had seen it and been duly impressed. He could see himself buying one. My elegiac feelings aside, I couldn't blame him; after all, he was running a men's store, not a museum.

I left Acappella feeling as if I'd accomplished something. Soon thereafter, I spoke with my parents. As occasionally happens when I tell them something slightly unusual, I was treated to a revelation. For example, when my wife-to-be and I had suggested that the wedding reception feature a buffet, my parents had met our proposal with desolate silence.

OPTION 2: THE SPREAD

Recommended suit: English three-button notch-lapel suit with side vents

Recommended knot: Windsor or double Windsor

Who should wear it: The wider-spread collar, which made its debut in England circa 1920, is best for men with narrow or oval faces. That means it demands a big knot. If you really want to make a statement, get a long tie (a.k.a. a "seven-fold") made from a thick material, and double or even triple that Windsor until your tie terminates with a commanding knot the size of a small fist.

You'll resemble: Jon Stewart, Jeremy Piven on *Entourage*, Wynton Marsalis, and Pierce Brosnan as 007

OPTION 3: THE BUTTON-DOWN

Recommended suit: Classic American two-button notch lapel with single vent

Recommended knot: Half Windsor

Who should wear it: This less formal collar—which was introduced in the United States in 1896 by Brooks Brothers—is the de facto choice for the dude who dons a suit simply because he must. It may seem like the height of convention today, but it was once the rebel's choice. According to Andy Gilchrist, author of *The Encyclopedia of Men's Clothes*, "before the button-down, most men's collars were stiff and detachable."

You'll resemble: Bill Gates, Ralph Lauren, and Jack Kerouac

My father clenched his jaw; my mother picked at her necklace, her eyes gleaming with tears. "Have you ever been to a Russian wedding with a buffet?" she asked. "It never happens," my father added. "Russians don't walk with plates," my mother concluded aphoristically, thereby acquainting me with a new facet of my culture.

My suit elicited a similar revelation, illustrative of the curious, paradoxical differences between the West and the former Soviet Union.

I was born in Riga, Latvia, in the spring of 1973, a drab, stagnant period in Soviet history. The misery of wars, famines, show trials, and mass deportations had given way to the more quotidian misery of shortages. It was a good news/bad news situation: One's odds of being sent to a gulag and one's odds of finding a decent salami were about the same. My father waited more than a decade to drive his own Lada; my aunt once camped out for a pair of boots; American blue jeans were a collective fantasy. Consumer items, particularly imported ones, were regarded

>>WEAR THIS, NOT THAT

The Shirt Cuff

What's up your sleeve can make or break a great suit. The key is knowing exactly how much of your hand to show.

Like launching a space shuttle or commenting on your girlfriend's body, matching shirt cuff to arm leaves virtually no margin for error. According to Andy Gilchrist, author of *The Encyclopedia of Men's Clothes*, one of the biggest fashion mistakes men make is sporting ill-fitting sleeves. But how to determine what's right? Rule of thumb: Perfect cuffs stop roughly at the base, where your hands meet your wrists. Assuming your suit is properly fitted, this will allow ¼ to ½ inch of shirtsleeve to extend beyond the jacket sleeve. Anything more and you're reenacting a notorious *Seinfeld* episode.

Too short: No cuff showing. Either the shirtsleeve is too short, the jacket sleeve is too long, or both. Bring both garments to your tailor and let him figure it out.

Too long: More than ½ inch of cuff showing. Either the shirtsleeve is too long, the jacket sleeve is too short, or both. Again, it's best to seek professional help.

On the mark: Showing ¼ to ½ inch of cuff.

with reverence and awe. An item's specific provenance mattered little as long as it was imported. The word "imported" (*im'portnii*) accrued totemic power and may very well have held claim to the title "most supremely flattering adjective in the Russian language." All of which leads me to a story about a very memorable incident in the lives of my parents.

One day my mother, herself a recent bride, chanced into a store and glimpsed a navy blue suit—on a rack. This already qualified as an exceptional occurrence. She drew near, inspected the suit (which was from Finland), and could scarcely believe her eyes. In her life she could not recall an instance of such great good fortune! Her euphoria, however, was immediately eclipsed by dreadful anxiety. She lacked the money to buy the suit. She despaired of leaving the store, fearing that when she returned, the suit would be gone. She ran to an aunt's house several blocks away, breathlessly explained her predicament, and was immediately loaned the requisite amount. She then rushed back and, to her jubilation, discovered that the suit was still there. She purchased it and brought it home to my father. My father tried it on and, as my mother had anticipated, it fit. (Here it helps to know that my father was not a hard man to fit. A dedicated sportsman, he maintained an athletic physique nearly until his death.) My parents were exceedingly happy.

This was both my father's first imported suit and his first off-the-rack suit.

Before this, what few suits my father had owned had all been made for him. The same held true for most Soviet men. If a man needed a suit, he secured a bolt of fabric and the services of a tailor. This posed its own complications, but it was still much easier than finding a ready-made garment. Hence the paradox. What in the West was a luxury, in Soviet Latvia was a banality. The highest mark of prestige in the Soviet Union was not a custom-made suit but something off-the-rack—preferably imported from Finland, Poland, Czechoslovakia, or some comparable fashion mecca. Most men, however, contented themselves with the handiwork of Soviet tailors. Which brings me to another story from my father's childhood.

When my father was 13, and then 14, he helped his father smuggle fabric. This was in Riga in the late 1940s, as the city and country were still recovering from the chaos and devastation of World War II. My grandfather was a notorious black marketer who, throughout his life, speculated in currency, precious metals, gems, and textiles. He was small, gaunt, and fierce. The authorities monitored his activities. Once, they brought him in for interrogation and tried to intimidate him. In response, my grandfather picked up a bulky ashtray and threatened to crack his interrogator's skull. He was released. In appearance and in temperament, my father didn't much resemble his own father, but he loved him and was intensely devoted to him.

To smuggle the fabric, my father and my grandfather would set out in the late evenings for warehouses and factories where my grandfather had his connections. The connections were managers or foremen who had distorted the inventory records to underrepresent the amount of fabric they had. My grandfather purchased the "surplus" and sold it to

⟩⟩WEAR THIS, NOT THAT

The Trouser Cuff

To cuff or not to cuff? Though neither option has ever gone entirely out of style, the right choice depends on your height and where you plan to play that day.

You should cuff your suit pants if . . . You're 5'10" or taller, you're a conservative dresser, or the forecast calls for rain. Why? According to Andy Gilchrist, author of *The Encyclopedia of Men's Clothes*, "the cuff was first adopted in the 1860s by British cricket players, who rolled up their pants to protect them from mud." Royalty and politicians followed suit, and the rest is fashion history. A standard cuff width is $1\frac{1}{2}$ inches and should always be hemmed straight across.

You should hem your suit pants if . . . You covet a more modern look, or you're 5'9" or shorter. A cuff, says *Men's Health* fashion director Brian Boyé, visually shrinks the leg, "making shorter men look even shorter." Formal dress trousers are another story. "They're never cuffed," says Gilchrist, "because as far as I know, there's rarely mud at formal occasions." For a subtler stylish look, have your tailor slant the bottoms so the hem is lower at the heel.

complicit tailors. The tailors used the material to sew suits, coats, or dresses for select customers willing to pay a premium. My grandfather's role was one of broker. He assumed risks others feared to assume. To move the material, my grandfather would wind it around my father's torso and waist and then cover him with an overcoat. The two of them then descended into the darkened streets.

Making a suit in the postwar Soviet Union was a perilous business. The MGB, precursor to the KGB, punished commercial crimes harshly, almost always with imprisonment. My grandfather brought my father along as cover, to appear less suspicious. He believed that a father and son would seem relatively innocuous, less likely to be stopped by the police. He proved to be correct. They were never stopped.

When my father told me the story, I asked him if he had been afraid. He shrugged in an abstract way. My mother asked him what he would have done had they been confronted. "What kind of question is that?" my father asked, without elaborating further. I understood that he would have done whatever my grandfather expected of him, including take the blame. It seemed to me that my grandfather had been reckless with my father's life. My father, of course, would never admit to any such thing. Many years later, after a vicious dispute and the resulting estrangement, my father nevertheless bristled if someone spoke an unkind word about my grandfather. I wasn't quite as forgiving. I felt no kinship with my grandfather. If I thought of him at all, it was only to marvel at his longevity. He lived to be 96. My father died at 70.

A month or so after I ordered my suit, I went to Acappella and picked it up. By then, in its finished form, it was no longer quite as compelling. It could have been any suit. To a certain extent, a suit is a suit is a suit. What had intrigued me, after all, was not getting a suit but getting a suit made. Now that it was made, it ceased to be a project and was instead an object—albeit an object that fit snugly through the shoulders and tapered subtly at the waist. As I walked out of the store with my suit, I could already feel its energy decaying, just like any other purchase. I imagined that some of the energy would remain residual, sustained—maybe indefinitely—by a few volts of sentiment.

I had a fairly clear idea of what my relationship would be to the suit.

I would wear it periodically, but mainly it would hang in my closet, where, now and again, I'd take note of it and be reminded of the dual ceremonies that brought it into existence: its own creation and my wedding. I would see replayed, filmlike, snippets of myself at Acappella, a still of Ulysses S. Grant at his tailor, and flashes of my wedding: vows, dancing, celebration. But things did not play out exactly according to this script. As I write this, the suit, in its blue garment bag, hangs in the closet, several feet behind my desk. If I turn my mind to it, I see— interspersed with Acappella, General Grant, and the wedding—my mother, a young bride, racing through the streets of Riga to buy a Finnish suit; and my father, 13 years old, an obedient son, bound tight under his overcoat, following my grandfather into the night.

YOUR CASUAL CLOTHING

WEED OUT THE WARDROBE WRECKERS

BY MATT BEAN

I'm standing in front of my closet staring at a tangled razor-wire mess of hangers. The paralysis seeps in slowly, like venom taking hold. It's 7:30 a.m., and somehow the simple task of selecting what to toss into a garment bag for a business trip has triggered a biological response meant to protect man from beast, not man from blazer. My heart pounds. The undershirt I just slipped on grows moist with sweat.

I shake my head and dive into the fray. Half an hour later, I've made my choices, and it means only one thing: During my week on the road, I'll constantly worry about whether I have everything I need, and if it all hangs together. It's not a huge deal, but not a small one, either.

When did something so simple—getting dressed—become so difficult?

If, like me, you've ever longed for the days when loincloths and body hair were haute couture, there's a reason. We're all victims of what researcher Barry Schwartz, PhD, calls the paradox of choice. The idea is quite simple: As consumers, we're bombarded by options, ill-equipped to make decisions, and, as a result, more dissatisfied than ever with everything from the clothing we wear to the cars we drive to the processed foods we consume.

"It's just getting worse and worse," says Schwartz. "Companies invent things for you to care about that never used to matter. So what if your distressed jeans were hand torn by grass-fed Australian cattle? But they'll keep telling you that it matters, and eventually, you'll believe them. And so you waste time deciding what to buy, and then once you get it home, you waste even more time deciding what to wear. And the more time you spend deciding what to wear, the less time you have to actually do something in your clothes."

Thankfully, Schwartz and fellow researchers have developed a simple set of rules for cutting through the confusion of any complicated decision-making event. They run against the grain of our choice-mad society—once you've had 200 cable channels, would you settle for basic?—but they work. Schwartz urges me to apply them to my problematic wardrobe. No matter what state your closet is in, this sort of garment guidance can help you look better in less time and feel better about the clothes you're wearing—and about yourself.

To start, all you'll need to do is figure out what not to wear. For me, that was easy. I hired a consultant.

Clinton Kelly is the cohost of the style-intervention show *What Not to Wear*, on TLC. His specialty is exactly the sort of sartorial evisceration my wardrobe needs: He ridicules unwitting victims into shaping up their style. Kelly is a *Men's Health* contributor, so I call for a consultation, and a week later, he's standing with me in front of my closet, asking me to forget the past.

"This is absolutely disgusting," he says as he dangles a shirt at arm's length over a pile of rumpled linen pants, bad ties, and ill-fitting suits. "You need to get rid of it, now."

The shirt he's holding like a soggy diaper is a faded, pit-stained Hagerstown Suns minor-league baseball shirt. My cousin Michael gave it to me the day I watched him spectacularly self-destruct on the mound 18 years ago. The shirt means a lot to me. Men shouldn't give up on their heroes, even if they are a little rough around the edges.

"Can't we just put it aside?" I plead.

This unholy experiment was supposed to reshuffle my tangle of hangers into a utilitarian closet that would help me look great with little effort—and, in the process, help you do the same. It wasn't supposed to rewrite my personal history.

"Listen, you have too much to worry about to keep a half-decent shirt in your wardrobe," says Kelly. "My rules are simple: If the stain hasn't come out yet, it's there to stay. If you haven't worn it in a year, you probably never will. And if it doesn't fit, you're better off using the space for something that does. Let's toss it and move on, and if you really decide you want it later, you can dig it out."

I cringe, and give in. One of the reasons we get lost in the clutter, I've learned, is that our wardrobes become archival rather than practical. A recent study shows that the average 29-year-old still has clothes that are more than 16 years old. Sometimes we just can't give up on the past, no matter how pathetic it was.

"Men are conditioned to look at garments as investments," says Mark-Evan Blackman, chairman of the menswear-design department at the Fashion Institute of Technology, in New York City. "But you can't think, 'Well, I paid $200 for these plaid pants, and therefore I'm going to keep them.' You can't think, 'Well, these clothes are part of me, they're like my kids, and I can't get rid of them.' Sometimes you just need to be told, 'Yes, but your kid is nasty, your kid is ugly, and your kid slobbers.' You just need to wake up."

So my Hagerstown Suns shirt is headed for the adoption line, evidently.

Lesson learned: The wardrobe should be an armory more than an orphanage. But what happens when its contents aren't ready for deployment?

"Do you actually wear this?" gasps Kelly, pulling a puke green shirt from the cluster in my closet. It's a French-cuffed number, fit for a man with arms half as long as mine. But my girlfriend says the color "makes my eyes pop," and that's not something to easily dismiss. I'd taken to rolling and rerolling the sleeves every 15 minutes to rein in the recalcitrant polyester.

"Well, yes," I admit. "It's one of my go-to shirts. I guess I was never willing to give up on it." And besides, who knows, maybe my arms will shrink.

Kelly's sneer underscores another important part of the purge process (and my underlying problem). Clothing, with its divergent cuts, colors, fabrics, styles, sizes, and fits, confronts us with an elaborate flowchart of decisions every time we get dressed. We're all bound to end up less happy because of the sheer number of forks in the road we're forced to consider.

The seminal study on the subject wasn't done on clothing, but on candy. A group of college students was asked to rate an array of 30 different chocolates, while another group was given six chocolates. Not only was the six-chocolate group more likely to enjoy the chocolates they tasted, they were also four times as likely to choose a box of chocolates offered in lieu of payment at the end of the study. Chocolate instead of money?

"When you have only six chocolates, it's easy to rule out a couple of them from the start—this one probably has nuts, this one's made from dark chocolate, and so on," says Mark Lepper, PhD, a researcher at Stanford University and the study's coauthor. "But not when you have 30. It's a remarkably powerful mechanism, restricting choice. There is no perfect choice. And the more potential decisions you have to make, the more compromises you'll make. The amount of potential dissatisfaction magnifies exponentially."

Let's apply this reasoning to clothing.

If your wardrobe consisted of a red jumpsuit and a blue jumpsuit, both cut from identical cloth, both the same size and style, your choice would be easy, right? Which color do you like better?

But add a variable—alter the red suit so it hugs your shoulders

▶▶SAVE THAT SWEATER

Moth-eaten or snagged sweaters don't have to die at the back of your closet. And put away your duct tape: Classic repair services can fix them right. Now's the time—before winter hits.

Knit Alteration & Design: (800) 662-5648 www.knitalteration.com: Burns, moth holes, unraveled fine knits—send them all in. Cost depends on the size of the hole and the knit.

Not Just Yarn: (802) 257-1145 notjustyarn.com: Located in Vermont, where they've always worn sweaters. One woman, Susan Vaiciulis, does all the repairs. She specializes in cashmere.

Knitwear Doctor: (800) 888-3459 knitweardoctor.com: They call it "reknitting"— taking yarn from an unobtrusive spot on the sweater to fix holes. They'll also fix sagging necklines (the sweater's, not your skin's).

Without a Trace: (800) 475-4922 withoutatrace.com: They specialize in reweaving (for small tears, holes, and burns), inweaving (for larger tears), and reknitting. They can restore leather, too.

better—and you're forcing a compromise. You'll go with the red one, say, because it fits better, but all you'll think about is how much you'd rather be wearing your favorite color, blue. Magnify this tug-of-war across all the hundreds of choices you make in front of your wardrobe every day and you can see how, even if you pick the perfect outfit, you'll never be perfectly satisfied.

For my odyssey, then, the second lesson is simple: Ditching the outright losers from my closet won't be enough—I'll also have to eliminate problems with the clothes I intend to keep.

I wheel a rolling garment bag of misfit shirts and suits to the midtown Manhattan quarters of tailor Wilfredo Rosario to manage my misfits. To Rosario, the bigger problem isn't to be found in the details of my clothing but in the depths of my brain.

"To me, an eighth of an inch might not mean anything. But to some guys, it can make or break a suit," says Rosario, scratching his head with a piece of tailor's chalk. "It's all mental. So my job isn't just to take care of your clothing. My job is to take care of you." He tugs on the shoulders of my suit, pats my back, and swivels me around to face the mirror. "You have to realize that it's all in your head."

His words fit me perfectly. They're the essence of the body-clothes connection. His tweaks and corrections to my wardrobe are, in fact, necessary adjustments to how I see myself. It makes the investment in a good scissor/needle man seem like a trifle.

I've spent far less time than I anticipated to become confident about what I want to wear and what looks good on me. And in clearing some of the clutter from the closet, I've been able to clear some of it from my head, to boot. So why not make the change official?

Why not rid myself of all this emotional baggage once and for all?

Back at home, I look into my newly efficient closet, then back at the reject pile. Everything is in its place. Well, almost. I reach down beneath all the rejected versions of me—the club-going, nylon-pants-wearing slickster; the mock-turtleneck-wearing cheeseball; the leather-jacket-clad disco porn star—and grab the gritty gray Hagerstown Suns T-shirt. I slip it on, then stuff everything else into a giant black garbage bag.

Nobody at the Salvation Army likes the Hagerstown Suns anyway.

THE COLOR ADVANTAGE

SHARPEN YOUR STYLE WITH SCIENCE

BY MATT BEAN; RESEARCH BY KYLE WESTERN

Fashion is of the moment; biology is not. That's why, among all the changing cuts, styles, and patterns in a man's wardrobe, there remains one constant: color. Our biological imperatives—among them social connections and reproduction—have been honing our hue smarts for hundreds of thousands of years, says Abby Calisch, PsyD, a psychology professor at Argosy University at Dallas and an expert on art therapy. The right color selections, she says, "can elicit emotions and feelings in those around us." In other words, if you choose your colors carefully, you can capture attention, soften up your conversational partners, or play hardball during a business negotiation. We pulled the research to find out just how to color your world.

Actor Jesse Spencer, who plays Dr. Robert Chase on the Fox series *House*, has a team of wardrobe pros dressing him as a healer who reserves his best bedside manner for his female patients. "I like wearing blue," he says. "It goes well with my eyes." He has the hang of it. Now it's your turn to play with matches.

ATTACK MODE: RED IS FOR THE AGGRESSOR

Red is a call to action. British researchers linked the color to high levels of aggression in a 2006 study of Olympic martial artists. "In many male primates, fish, and birds, redness of the skin correlates with testosterone," says study coauthor Robert Barton, PhD. "Red triggers an unconscious appraisal of the opponent as more dominant." How to wield the color wisely? "Temper it with neutral colors," says *Men's Health* fashion director Brian Boyé. Another, more subtle option: Choose a red accessory as a reminder of your dominance.

COOLING TREND: SET YOURSELF TO STUN

Blue works well anywhere, from a boardroom to a barbecue. But it's not just a laid-back utility infielder, according to researchers at the University of Utah. Color-sensing structures in her eyes preferentially pick out the hue and forward the info on a more direct path to her brain. Choose a blue that matches the formality of your event. The more buttoned up, the darker the hue. "It's the foundation of many key looks," says Boyé. Accessorizing properly will accentuate the effect. "Brown dress shoes, rather than black, will help a navy suit really pop from afar. It's how the Italians do it, after all."

PEACE TIME: PERFECT THE CHILL-OUT

Pastels can moderate aggressive behavior, even in prison inmates, according to a seminal 1979 study done at the Institute for Biosocial Research, in Tacoma, Washington. So think what they'll do for you.

▶▶DETAIL YOUR DIGITS

Unkempt hands and feet can send women running. Three steps to a softer touch.

Step 1: Think straight. Start with a simple horizontal clip across each nail. "Cutting at an angle trains the nail to grow that way," says Denise Vitiello, director of the fitness center and spa at the Mandarin Oriental hotel in New York City. Round off corners with a medium-grit emery board—never a harsh metal file—filing in one direction only.

Step 2: Thin your skin. Massage the pads of your palms and the sides of your heels and feet with an exfoliating scrub, using firm, circular strokes with your thumbs. This breaks down thickened areas of skin, which can develop into corns or fissures, says Cary Zinkin, DPM, a spokesperson for the American Podiatric Medical Association.

Step 3: Kill the fungi. Dry your dogs, then hit them with a cold-air blast from a hair dryer to evaporate any remaining moisture, which could harbor the fungi that cause athlete's foot. Then slather a thick moisturizer on your hands and feet after you leave the shower. "Everyone forgets the feet," says Dr. Zinkin. "But they're even more important to moisturize because of all the rubbing in the shoes."

"They're perfect for mediating situations or making a good first impression," says fashion expert Laura Siebold. "Just make sure you don't look like a bouquet." Wear pastels to casual outdoor events or use them to take the edge off a more somber suit ensemble. Even subtle pastel accents make a difference.

GRAY AREAS: PROJECT MYSTERY, NOT MISERY

A Cornell University study found that professional teams with predominantly black uniforms were perceived to be more aggressive than teams wearing lighter colors; they were also penalized more. "It makes you look slick," says Joe Lupo, co-owner of Visual Therapy, an image-and-style consulting service. "And sometimes that's not the best impression to give." A dark gray suit might help silence the penalty whistles. Pair it with a colorful shirt. "You have to warm it up," says Foley. Save your darkest colors for nighttime, when they'll blend better with surroundings.

SKIN GAME: BLEND IN TO STAND OUT

Shade-savvy dressers make sure each piece of clothing not only matches its neighbors but also complements the body palette nature gave them. "Color reflects against your skin, and a differentiated look will prevent you from appearing washed out," says Julie Foley, an image consultant in Boston. Foley adds another wrinkle: eye color. Green and blue tones complement lighter eye colors; browns and blacks, darker eyes. Let your skin tone determine the intensity—the lighter your skin, the paler the palette of your shirts. Use pants and jackets as a frame; contrast them with your hair and shirt colors for maximum effect.

IMAGE UPGRADES

LIFE'S REWARDS OFTEN COME AT A STEEP PRICE. CUT COSTS WITHOUT CUTTING CORNERS

BY LUKE COLLINS

Rich guys don't stay that way by buying bling. Spotting value—whether you're a bloodthirsty corporate raider or just a guy with a few bucks in his pocket and a yen for the finer things in life—ultimately makes any purchase more satisfying. "When you find something you love at a price that's less than somebody else might pay, it adds to the whole experience," says Jean Chatzky, financial editor for the *Today* show and author of *Pay It Down!* "It's a game of one-upmanship; it feels good to feel smarter." Here's how to spend less on life's biggest luxuries, so you can afford more and more of them.

DRIVE THE HOTTEST CAR IN THE HOOD

James Bond had an Aston Martin DB5. Steve McQueen, a 1968 Mustang. You have . . . a Kia? Your salvation: a classic sports car, says Joe Lorio, senior editor at *Automobile* magazine. "It looks really cool, and nobody knows you paid the same as somebody who just bought a new Ford Explorer." Lorio's ultimate vintage ride: a Mercedes 230, 250, or 280 SL built between 1964 and 1971 (about $35,000). Want something more recent? Look on eBay Motors or www.cars.com for an older version of a model that hasn't changed much. "You'll get the same performance and the same head-snapping recognition, without the higher price tag," says Lorio.

Our picks: a mid-to-late-1990s BMW 328is with manual transmission (about $8,000) or a late-'90s Jaguar XK8 (about $25,000). Spooked by potentially expensive repair costs? Check out the swoopy lines of a Nissan 300ZX built between 1990 and 1996, or the two-door Lexus

SC400 coupe from the same period (about $15,000)—both have impeccable mechanical histories.

GAMBLE LIKE A HIGH ROLLER

Play your cards right and you could stretch a short stack of chips into a night's worth of entertainment. "Look at the house edge and the speed of the game," says Frank Scoblete, author of *Beat the Craps out of the Casinos*. "How many games you play per hour and how many decisions you have to make can determine how fast the casino's edge adds up." Blackjack might give the dealer only a 0.5 percent statistical advantage, but you'll play as many as 100 hands per hour. Roulette is slow-paced, but the dealer has a whopping 5.26 percent advantage.

Scoblete's advice: Join a packed blackjack table so the dealer can't churn through cards as fast, or belly up to a craps table, which offers some of the best odds in the casino. Forget about the patchwork quilt of betting options and lay down $6 "place" bets on both the 6 and the 8. Whenever someone rolls either of those two numbers, you'll win $7 for every $6 you wager. Odds dictate that will happen 10 times out of 36 rolls. "You're getting a lot of action at the table without being involved in all the decisions," says Scoblete. "That's a lot of entertainment for your money."

START THE ULTIMATE WINE CELLAR

Wine worth savoring shouldn't sap your savings. "You just have to find new regions and undiscovered wines," says Paul Lang, owner of New York City wine-events group A Casa. "As soon as something is covered by the media, the prices skyrocket." Beat the hordes by trolling wine blogs—we like www.corkjester.com and www.vinography.com—for under-the-radar picks, and by cultivating a relationship with your local provider. You're looking for three things: First, unexpected home runs. "You might not think to pick up a wine from Greece or Uruguay, which is exactly why you should," says Jeffery Lindenmuth, owner of www.pawinepicks.com. Second, up-and-coming hot spots. "Focus your gaze on emerging regions," says Joshua Wesson, chairman and executive wine director of Best Cellars. Spanish wines have buzz, but avoid the already-hot Rioja region and concentrate on nearby La Mancha, Jumilla, and Toro, for example. And third, trickle-down quality. Pick up a second-label wine from a solid producer—like Hawk Crest instead of the more expensive Stag's Leap, from Stag's Leap Wine Cellars, in Napa, California. "Wineries create these brands to use up the grapes that aren't quite good enough for their best wines," says Lindenmuth. "They're an especially great buy in the best years, when an abundance of fantastic grapes carries over into the lower-priced wines."

COLLECT RARE ART

A Picasso can cost millions, because it's one-of-a-kind. Sacrifice scarcity, but not quality, and anyone can afford fine art. "If it's a good example of a very good artist's work, then it's a safe investment," says Cary Leibowitz, a vice president at auction house Christie's. Prints or lithographs from established artists, including Louise Nevelson and James Whistler, average $2,000, and works from emerging artists can be even cheaper. Three hot spots, according to Robin Cembalest, executive editor of www.artnews.com: Affordable Art Fair (www.aafnyc.com), which sells works ranging from $100 to $5,000; Artists Space gallery (www.artistsspace.org), a collective that features print works from up-and-coming artists; and the art magazine *Parkett*.

WOW HER WITH CHEAP FLOWERS

Dropping $70 on a dozen roses isn't just expensive; it's obvious. Calla lilies or orchids are more exotic, but an arrangement of tropical leaves is an even better alternative. They can deliver the same aesthetic punch for a third of the cost. "They'll have the same long, elegant lines and striking colors, the hallmarks of high-end arrangements," says party planner David Tutera, who has thrown flower-laden bashes for the Rolling Stones, Elton John, and Matthew McConaughey.

Any serious florist should have a range of varieties, depending on the season, but a good start would be magnolia leaves, pampas plumes, and monstera leaves, tied together with raffia or twine. It'll make a statement. Bonus: They'll cost half as much (around $25) and last twice as long (up to 2 weeks) as most flowers.

EAT AT FIVE-STAR RESTAURANTS

Taking culinary advice from an expense-account-wielding food critic is like soliciting gas-mileage advice from Halliburton. Instead, turn to the people who understand value best: devoted foodies who shell out precious greenbacks for every morsel they consume. The boom in foodie Web sites, such as www.egullet.org and www.chowhound.com, means instant access to legions of dedicated gastronomes, quietly uncovering the country's best restaurant bargains. Whether you're in search of roadside barbecue in rural North Carolina or an omakase sushi feast in Tokyo, log on, search the forums, and if your question hasn't already been answered (it probably has), start a new thread. Within days, the culinary nerds of the region will have rendered a list for you.

"Instead of getting just one opinion, you tap into a range of knowledge and experience," says Marlene Newell, chief administrative officer of www.egullet.org. These sites also track the world's up-and-coming culinary stars, so if a young sous-chef has left a revered temple, they'll let you know where he or she surfaces, and you may be able to taste all those delicious secrets at a fraction of the original price.

THROW THE PARTY OF THE YEAR

Hosting a top-notch, low-cost soiree means downsizing your menu. "The guests should be raving about your dynamite mojitos or guacamole the next day, not trying to remember which of the 19 hors d'oeuvres they liked best," says Tutera, author of *Big Birthdays*. For a signature drink, premix a vodka-based cocktail from www.webtender.com using midshelf booze. "You know those guys who swear they can tell Grey Goose from Gordon's with one swig? They're full of it," says Lauren Purcell, coauthor of *Cocktail Parties, Straight Up!* Another tip: Find a wine retailer who's willing to knock 10 percent off the cost of a case of mixed wine, says Tutera.

For an appetizer, try bite-size comfort food with an upscale twist. Chef John Greeley, of New York City's 21 Club restaurant, uses this simple recipe to make about 25 finger-size meat treats: Mix together 8 ounces of regular ground sirloin and 8 ounces of top round with 2 ounces of dry-aged sirloin, then add 2 tablespoons of rendered duck fat or shortening, 2 tablespoons of sliced fresh chives, and half a cup of chopped white onion. Season with 1 tablespoon of ground black pepper and 1 teaspoon each of thyme, cayenne pepper, paprika, and fine-ground Indian coriander. Broil melon ball–size patties until brown and brush with olive oil before adding a pinch of Cheddar cheese. Serve on toasted 1-inch circles of white bread (use an overturned shot glass as a cutting template) and top with a dollop of ketchup and a sprinkle of chives.

CONVERT YOUR HOME INTO A CASTLE

High-end homes house more than just $9,000 end tables. "What really makes an impression is creating the right sort of ambience," says designer Thomas O'Brien. The quickest fix? Lighting. Ditch ceiling lights, which cast harsh shadows on faces and objects in the room, in favor of reflective lighting—torchieres, desk lamps, or floor-mounted can lamps. "I use as much lamplight as possible," says O'Brien. "It provides a soft, comfortable, easy light that's flattering." Keep bulb wattage to 40, look for a soft pink or peach tint, and mount lamps below standing height to avoid a spotlight effect.

BUILD YOUR OWN HOME THEATER

Adding wattage to your home-entertainment setup doesn't have to mean taking on a second mortgage. Most off-brand LCD and plasma manufacturers use the same parts, panels, and even factories that their more pedigreed shelf-mates use, meaning you can buy a near-Sony-quality picture for a pittance. "Most no-name sets offer a good enough picture quality for most people, and sometimes very good picture quality," says David Katzmaier, CNET's TV editor. For example, LCD panels from Sam's Club mainstay Vizio actually come from upmarket TV maker LG. For maximum picture for the price, we like the Maxent MX-50X3 50-inch plasma (we found it as low as $2,400) and the Vizio L32HDTV 32-inch LCD (as low as $1,000).

Still want the name-brand luster? Most major manufacturers and retailers dump overstocked and reconditioned gear on outlet sites, with markdowns as high as 60 percent. We found a new Philips 32-inch LCD for $800 (at www.outlet.philips.com, regularly $1,075) and a

Zenith 5.1-channel, 300-watt home-theater system for $125 (at Circuit City's outlet, regularly $230). The finishing touch: Expand your film library by swapping unwanted movies at www.peerflix.com, which matches you with others for by-mail trades—at only $1 per trade.

VACATION LIKE A CELEBRITY

Living large abroad on a small budget takes lateral thinking. If you can't afford Paris or Prague, try Poland instead. "Kraków is just as beautiful and just as bustling with music and outdoor entertainment, and it hasn't been killed by its own popularity," says Frommer's Travel Guides scion Pauline Frommer. Travel in summer and stay on the city's most beloved street in a building dating from the 14th century, the Hotel Pod Roza (www.hotel.com.pl/podroz; doubles from $205 a night).

If you want sun and sand, avoid St. Barts and Anguilla. "Margarita Island, off the coast of Venezuela, is unspoiled compared with its Caribbean neighbors," says Frommer. "And the Venezuelan currency is so low, it's cheap for Americans." Summer hurricane season is always cheapest—and riskiest; double rooms at the massive LagunaMar (www.lagunamar.com.ve) begin at around $145 a night.

For snow fun, ditch Vail in favor of Canada's Whistler—packages at www.whistlerblackcomb.com are reasonable all year, and are even cheaper as spring approaches. "At Whistler, the mountain is so high, you're going to have good snow right into spring," says Frommer. Travel site www.biddingfortravel.com can help you make the most of travel-auction Web sites www.priceline.com and www.luxurylink.com, says Susan Stellin, author of *How to Travel Practically Anywhere*. You could save 15 percent.

KNOW WHAT YOU LIKE

Whoever coined the phrase "easy on the eyes" may have been onto something. In a study in the journal *Psychological Science,* 68 people viewed an abstract image on a computer screen. Researchers then showed them similar images and asked them to rate their appeal. Participants judged the patterns that were closest to the original as the most attractive. These findings may relate to perceptions of human beauty.

"What you like is a function of what you've been trained to like," says lead researcher Piotr Winkielman, PhD. "A stimulus becomes attractive if it falls into the average of what you've seen and is therefore simple for your brain to process."

C A BETTER SMILE

It's the all-purpose antioxidant, and now it doubles as a toothbrush: Vitamin C may reduce plaque and tartar formation, according to a study published in the *European Journal of Oral Science.* Researchers asked 30 people to chew gum—either a plain sugar-free piece or one fortified with 60 milligrams of vitamin C—every day for 3 months. They found that the people who chewed the fortified gum had 33 percent less tartar—a product of plaque buildup—on their teeth than their peers did.

Think of vitamin C as an acid bath for your bicuspids. "Vitamin C, a.k.a. ascorbic acid, stops plaque from sticking to teeth," says lead author Peter Lingstrom, DDS, PhD. Vitaball chewing gum, which is like a low-potency multivitamin, contains 60 mg vitamin C per piece.

FESS UP

Tell your plastic surgeon about the herbal supplements you're taking, or you may find a surprise in the mirror. Glucosamine and chondroitin (for joint pain), the immunity booster echinacea, and other herbal supplements may cause complications in plastic-surgery patients, according to the journal *Plastic and Reconstructive Surgery*.

DRESS DOWN

Wearing designer denim to work is a genius move all around. Researchers at the University of Wisconsin found that people who wore jeans to the office logged more steps throughout the day than they did on days when they were dressed in business attire. The scientists think that increased feelings of comfort made the employees more apt to be active.

Suit wearers

Before lunch 3,023 steps

During lunch 762 steps

After lunch 2,382 steps

Total 6,167 steps (2.91 miles)

Jeans wearers

Before lunch 3,331 steps

During lunch 821 steps

After lunch 2,566 steps

Total 6,718 steps (3.18 miles)

All that extra walking can benefit you in many ways. Here are just a few:

SHARPER VISION: Leaving your desk for just 5 minutes gives your eyes some much-needed recovery time from the strain caused by staring at your computer screen, according to a study in the *American Association of Occupational Health Nurses Journal.*

A HAPPIER STAFF: Employees feel better about their bosses when they see them face-to-face, rather than communicate by e-mail, according to researchers at Claremont Graduate University.

DISEASE-FREE ARTERIES: Socializing at the office could save your life. Johns Hopkins University researchers recently found that isolated employees are more likely to develop, and die of, cardiovascular disease.

DRESS FOR COMFORT

On days when you don't have to dress to impress, clothe for cognition. A Harvard study found that dressing comfortably can boost brainpower. In a study of 88 students, those wearing sweats earned higher marks on cognitive-ability tests than those in suits. "We had assumed that looking good made people feel good and helped them perform better," says lead author Richard Bell, PhD. Instead, discomfort may distract the brain and make it harder to retrieve information. Luckily, designers like Armani and Theory offer wider-legged pants made of a cotton/Lycra blend that are almost as comfortable as sweats.

SAVE YOUR SKIN

You don't drink lead-laden water, so why wash with it? Study results, published first in *Men's Health*, found skin-sabotaging metals in 28 U.S. cities' water supplies, says New York University professor Dennis Gross, MD, who analyzed the data. Clean up your water with a National Science Foundation–certified filter.

Accumulated deposits are photoactivated (energized) by the sun and can cause DNA mutations that may lead to skin cancer.

EAT MORE CHOCOLATE

Chocolate used to be a skin-problem scapegoat. But German scientists have discovered that the antioxidants in chocolate may protect skin from sun damage and even improve its appearance. The researchers found that when people drank a cocoa beverage high in compounds called flavonols every day for 12 weeks, their skin exhibited 25 percent less damage from ultraviolet (UV) rays.

Antioxidants may absorb UV light and prevent inflammation, says study author Wilhelm Stahl, PhD. They may also boost bloodflow throughout the skin, improving texture. Although participants drank the flavonol equivalent of 22 Hershey's Kisses daily, smaller doses over a lifetime may yield similar results, says Stahl. Try Mars CocoaVia chocolate bars, the only brand that guarantees a high level of antioxidants.

WANT A NEW DRUG

Frequent tanning can hook people like a drug, according to a Wake Forest University study. When researchers gave 16 tanning-salon regulars either a placebo or 15 milligrams of naltrexone—a substance-abuse medication—for 2 weeks, those taking the drug became 66 percent less interested in tanning. What's more, several of them also suffered jitters and nausea—signs of mild opiate withdrawal that occur when addicts take naltrexone.

UV light may increase the release of endorphins, activating the same brain mechanism that causes morphine addiction. Wean yourself by working out; exercise also provides an endorphin hit. And for a safe suntan, try St. Tropez Bronzing Mist Spray ($35).

GROOMING KIT

The Norelco 6 in 1 Professional Grooming Kit trims head hair, beards, mustaches, nose hair, ear hair, and eyebrows. No follicle is safe. ($30. www.norelco.com)

45 BRAUN 360 COMPLETE ELECTRIC SHAVER 8995

Most electric shavers overpromise and underdeliver, leaving your mug peppered with forgotten hairs and half-harvested stubble no better than a 5 o'clock shadow. This one actually makes good on the hype, thanks to a "powercomb" feature that brushes flat-lying hairs away from the skin and into the path of its blades. It nabbed our pesky neck scruff that others ignored. ($220. www.braun.com)

COLOR-CHANGING CLOTHES

Science may soon streamline your wardrobe. Researchers at the University of Connecticut have developed a T-shirt fabric that can change colors to match your preferences or the pants you're pairing it with. Electrochromic polymers, which contain electrons that absorb different wavelengths of light to create different colors and patterns, are woven into the textile. By using a small battery-powered controller, wearers can adjust the high-tech tees themselves, or plug them into a digital camera to display a preset pattern.

ZIT ZAPPER

Dermatologists at Harvard have developed a device that may put an end to acne. It's called a free-electron laser, and it can destroy parts of the oil-producing sebaceous glands without harming the skin's upper layers. As a result, excess oil won't plug pores and become infected by bacteria. Human trials on the pimple blaster are expected to begin soon.

HAIR GROWTH MEDICINE

Procter & Gamble has teamed up with the drug company Curis to create a new medication for male-pattern baldness. The topical treatment will stimulate a genetic pathway known as Hedgehog (named for the fruit fly species in which it was discovered) to encourage dormant hair follicles to function again. Preliminary animal studies have been successful, and tests on hairless humans are next.

SCENTS AND SENSIBILITY

HERE'S HOW TO WIELD FIVE WINNING SCENTS

1. **KEEP IT CLOSE:** Your "scent circle" should extend no farther than your reach. If someone outside that zone can name what cologne you're wearing, you've overdone it. "Too much of an odorant stimulates the same nerve in the brain that makes you cry when you're cutting onions," says Alan Hirsch, MD, neurological director of the Smell & Taste Treatment and Research Foundation. Be subtle: "Three to five sprays should be adequate," says Rochelle Bloom, president of the Fragrance Foundation, a fragrance-industry organization. "Just enough to give off a whiff of the scent."

2. **CHECK YOUR OIL:** Ask for a take-home sample of a new fragrance to see how your oils change the way it smells. "The oil glands put out several different types of oils that interact with the fragrance," says Wilma Bergfeld, MD, head of dermatological research at the Cleveland Clinic. Your skin's natural lube can also affect how long a scent lasts. Oilier skin tends to trap a fragrance, helping it endure, while dry skin might require a quick refresher before the day is done.

3. **SKIP STINKY MEALS:** Certain foods, especially garlic, olive oil, onions, and curry, exude strong smells through your sweat glands. "The pungent ones have the most specific odors," says Dr. Bergfeld. Don't try to offset the effect with more cologne; it'll create an even more noxious combination. Her advice is to skip the stinky stuff for 24 hours before an event at which you want to be olfactorily attractive.

4. **GIVE HER A WHIFF:** Shop for cologne with a woman, preferably a younger one. "Women have a better sense of smell than men, and that sense worsens for both genders as you age," says Dr. Hirsch. "So women might pick up notes in a scent that a man won't get."

5. **HIT THE HOT SPOTS:** Aim for areas of the body where the blood vessels are closer to the surface, which helps warm the skin so the alcohol in the cologne can evaporate into the air. Start with the pulse points at your wrists and neck and dab a bit behind your ears, says Bloom. You can also spritz some on your ankles. "Fragrance rises, so if you put it lower, it will linger longer," she says.

BURNING QUESTIONS

I lost a ton of weight and now nothing fits. Should I have my clothes tailored, or buy new?

Hit the mall. "You can tailor down one size, but you can't tailor beyond that," says Elena Castaneda, a Manhattan-based image consultant. Anything more than that and the styling is lost. Moreover, your old clothes "carry negative connotations of when you were heavy," says Marcy Carmack, a stylist and the creator of San Francisco's Chic Wardrobe Solutions.

It can't hurt to take a couple of your best pieces to a tailor to see what he can do. But toss everything else and show off the results of your hard work. For instance, trade in pleated, high-rise pants for ones with a slimmer, flat-front, midrise fit. Watch how shirts fit your armpits; they should come in close instead of tenting out toward your breastbone. It's fine to try out some trends, but stock up on classics—simple, well-fitting shirts and trousers. If you still have some pounds left to drop, Carmack suggests buying as few items as possible and bargain hunting. But splurge on one item, like a suede or leather jacket.

When is it okay to use the jacket of my navy suit as a blazer?

When you're wearing blue jeans. That's it. Coupling tailored suit jackets with more rugged denim always has a stylish effect, dressing up the jeans rather than slumming down the suit. Pairing your navy suit jacket with anything else, however—especially dress pants in a different color—will look like you selected both items from a bargain-basement clearance rack. Don't confuse suit jackets with blazers, though; blazers are designed to be more versatile, and thus can be worn with jeans, chinos, flannels, or even a kilt, if that's your thing.

I goof up whenever I try to iron. What's the key?

Steam, the wonder vapor. If you just let a steam iron huff and puff around a shirt on a hanger, you'll erase lots of wrinkles without risking hot steel on defenseless fabric. But you should learn to iron: You'll find a rare satisfaction in this skill.

Moisten your clothes first, says Steve Boorstein, author of *The Clothing Doctor's Ultimate Guide to Shopping & Caring for Clothing.* Dry wrinkles are set wrinkles. Use a spray bottle or a damp sponge.

Upgrade. Cheap irons leak. Try Rowenta's Professional DX8800 ($100, www.linensandthings.com). It shoots steam from the back for one-pass pressing.

Place aluminum foil under the cover of the ironing board. It'll speed things up by deflecting heat upward, so you're hitting the cloth from both sides.

Line up your pants crease or shirtsleeve on the board's edge to reduce the chance of ironing in a crooked crease.

Try homemade starch: 1 tablespoon of cornstarch dissolved in 2 cups of water in a spray bottle.

Ignore the phone. Distractions lead to burns. Don't get confused and answer the iron.

1. Begin with the inside and outside of the collar. Start at the tips and work your way to the back.

2. Do cuffs well—high visibility.

3. Slide the shoulder onto the end of the board.

4. Do the sleeves. Start at the cuff opening, then move to the top.

5. Iron the body. Start at the top and go down. The back is low priority; it'll wrinkle anyway.

6. Slide the tip of the iron between the buttons. You're done!

What shoes should I own?

Here's your lineup: two pairs of lace-ups, in brown and black; loafers; a pair of boots; and a hybrid. These will take you anywhere, says *Men's Health* fashion director Brian Boyé.

First, pull all your shoes out of the closet. Toss any with worn heels, cracked leather, chunky heels, or square toes. Polish the survivors with either cream or oil-based polish, and repeat every 2 to 3 weeks; it helps shoes last longer and "makes you more likely to wear a pair you haven't looked at for months," Boyé says. And invest in cedar shoe trees, which wick away moisture and keep the shoes in shape. Sand the cedar every year to refresh its power.

PERCENTAGE OF MEN WHO HAVE HAD A PROFESSIONAL SHOESHINE: 33

BLACK DRESS SHOES: Choose something clean and simple; it's more versatile. Stylish now means a bit elongated and narrow in the foot. Wear with: Black or gray suits or trousers; if they have a high polish, with a tuxedo. Bass ($95. www.bassshoes.com)

HYBRID: This should be your weekend shoe. Do not make your running shoes do double duty. This moisture-wicking pair washes up easily. Wear with: Khakis or jeans. Timberland Koschuta Sport oxfords ($90. www.timberland.com)

BROWN DRESS SHOES: Opt for medium brown instead of reddish or dark brown. Wear with: Brown, olive, gray (yes, gray), and navy suits or trousers, or to dress up jeans. Johnston & Murphy Nebel Moc Toe ($140. johnstonandmurphy.com)

LOAFERS: Your go-anywhere option, for weekends, workdays, or travel. Wear with: Khakis or trousers at work, jeans when relaxing. These are dressy enough for a suit.

Cole Haan Collection Air Marley Venetian ($300. www.colehaan.com)

BOOTS: You need something rugged for hikes, crummy weather, or a boost of testosterone. Wear with: Jeans (a look women love); cargos and cords are okay, too. Snowstorm? Rock them with a suit and tie. Cole Haan Air Mosby Lace boots ($225. www.colehaan.com)

Should I upgrade the old stuff in my medicine cabinet?

First off, don't call it a medicine cabinet. No drugs should be stored there, over-the-counter or prescription. The bathroom's heat and moisture cause medication to deteriorate and lose potency, says Jackson Como, PharmD, director of the University of Alabama at Birmingham's drug-information service.

Instead, keep the cabinet stocked with toiletries and first-aid products. These go-to players still have game: Band-Aids and Neosporin (for cuts) and Lamisil (for athlete's foot). Then add the following products to your roster.

CREST PRO-HEALTH TOOTHPASTE: A study in a dental journal found that this product performed better than other brands in relieving gum inflammation and removing tartar and plaque. ($4. www.crest.com)

GLIDE DEEP CLEAN FLOSS: Research shows that people who added flossing (using Glide's shred-resistant Deep Clean) to their brushing regimen saw a 38 percent decrease in gingival bleeding in just 2 weeks. ($4.50. www.cvs.com)

LAB SERIES FOR MEN INSTANT MOISTURE GEL: Three-quarters of the population gets dry skin at some point in the winter, research found. This lightweight, oil-free formula is absorbed quickly by the skin. ($26. www.labseriesformen.com)

OPTI-FREE REPLENISH CONTACT-LENS SOLUTION: People typically wear contacts for 13 hours a day. Lab testing found that Opti-Free keeps them moisturized for 14 hours. Plus, six of 10 optometrists recommend this brand. ($5. www.optifree.com)

ORAL-B VITALITY ELECTRIC TOOTHBRUSH: Its oscillating and rotating brush head moves 7,600 times a minute. Your hand brush: 260 times. This is a stripped-down version of Oral B's Professional Care model, which is $100 more. ($20. www.oralb.com)

SKINCEUTICAL ANTIOXIDANT LIP REPAIR: This stick reduces the free radicals caused by sunlight, and toxins that contribute to photoaging, says Jennifer Kim, MD, a dermatology professor at UCLA. ($30. www.skinstore.com)

CHLORASEPTIC DEFENSE DAILY HEALTH STRIPS: Lozenges merely increase saliva and mucus production to combat throat irritation. These dissolving strips contain vitamin C and zinc—proven immunity boosters. ($4. www.chloraseptic.com)

Do razors with four blades really work better than those with three?

Surprisingly, yes. Although the multiblade razors made by Schick (four-blade Quattro) and Gillette (five-blade Fusion) smack of marketing gimmicks, there's some good science behind them, says Bruce Katz, MD, professor of dermatology at the Mount Sinai School of Medicine. At least, that's what he found in a recent study of four- and five-blade razors at the Juva Skin and Laser Center, in New York City.

"Multiple blades allow the hairs to be cut with less friction," explains Katz, adding that swiping once with five blades is the equivalent of taking five passes with one blade, without the resulting irritation. But five blades are where the benefits stop. "If you go to six blades, you'll see minimal improvement," says Katz. In short, don't waste your money if Schick ever comes out with a "Sei" razor.

Is using mouthwash just as good as flossing?

Nope. "There's simply no substitute for flossing," says Charles H. Perle, DMD, a spokesman for the American Academy of General Dentistry and a dentist in Jersey City, New Jersey. Mouthwash with fluoride and essential oils helps prevent tooth decay and plaque, but it can't dislodge the food and bacteria crammed between your teeth the way floss can.

As for the age-old question, waxed or unwaxed? A study showed no difference in effectiveness. Use what you like. But use it.

Can laser combs help prevent or reverse hair loss?

Save your money. As yet, there's no good scientific data to show conclusively that laser combs help regrow lost hair—or keep it from falling out of your scalp in the first place.

I'm going gray. Can I slow it down without dye?

Probably not. "There is no known method of preventing or slowing down the graying process," says Laurence Meyer, PhD, a professor of dermatology at the University of Utah. That said, a new study found that oxidative stress is a factor in graying—so eating foods rich in antioxidants (such as fruit and beans) might help slow the process.

Too late for you? Try Just for Men, suggests Dana Rogalski, of the American Board of Certified Haircolorists. According to the manufacturer, its colors are less vibrant (containing fewer red tones) than women's dyes, and work they faster because they don't strip away natural color before applying the new color.

Warning: The dye may appear darker in your hair than it is on the box, says Rogalski.

There's better news on the distant horizon. Harvard researchers have connected graying to the die-off of adult stem cells underneath the scalp. These stem cells produce cells called melanocytes that give hair its pigment. If scientists can pinpoint the trigger that starts the die-off, a surefire treatment could emerge.

INDEX

Underscored page references indicate boxed text.